Supported

Your Guide to Birth and Baby

Kristin Revere, MM, CED, NCS
Alyssa Veneklase, CED-PIC, NCS

Praeclarus Press. LLC
www.PraeclarusPress.com

Praeclarus Press, LLC
2504 Sweetgum Lane
Amarillo, Texas 79124 USA
806-367-9950
www.PraeclarusPress.com

DISCLAIMER

The information contained in this publication is advisory only and is not intended to replace sound clinical judgment or individualized patient care. The author disclaims all warranties, whether expressed or implied, including any warranty as the quality, accuracy, safety, or suitability of this information for any particular purpose.

ISBN: 978-1-946665-72-0

Cover Design: Ken Tackett
Copyediting: Chris Tackett
Layout and Design: Nelly Murariu

Contents

Foreword

As someone who has dedicated my professional life to supporting expectant mothers and their families in their journey through pregnancy and beyond, I can confidently attest to the importance of having a comprehensive, knowledgeable, and compassionate guide during this transformative time.

Supported: Your Guide to Birth and Baby, written by the highly experienced Gold Coast Doulas, is exactly the resource that families have long needed. This insightful and supportive book, much like the important work of a doula, encourages you to feel confident, informed, and well-prepared as you navigate this life-changing journey.

Just as each pregnancy and birth is unique, so too should be the team of experts assembled to support and guide an expectant mother. The guidance provided in this book ensures that women and their families can understand their available options for support, ultimately empowering them to make the best decisions tailored to their needs.

The comprehensive layout of the book, from early pregnancy to the postpartum period, mirrors the course of the pregnancy journey itself, thus making the information easily accessible and applicable. Each chapter provides practical advice, personal stories, and expert observations that combine to form a rich tapestry of shared wisdom and insight.

What sets *Supported* apart from other resources is its authors' commitment to inclusivity, recognizing and respecting the diversity of the birthing community. They skillfully weave together personal experiences, evidence-based research, and their vast professional knowledge in a manner that speaks to all readers. This approach aligns perfectly with the values of Informed Pregnancy Media, where we believe that informed decisions are the cornerstone of empowering birth experiences.

An especially commendable aspect of *Supported* is its integration of insight from various experts, offering readers a well-rounded and multifaceted perspective on maternity care. By incorporating a diverse range of wisdom, knowledge, and advice, the authors foster an inclusive and comprehensive resource that caters to the unique needs of every expectant mother. As a chiropractor, I've seen first-hand how vital it is for expectant mothers to feel physically balanced and comfortable throughout their pregnancy. The wisdom shared by Heidi McDowell in this book beautifully complements this goal, and I believe readers will find her advice invaluable.

In essence, this book is akin to having a wise and comforting doula at your side throughout your pregnancy journey, providing reassurance and guidance every step of the way. It is a resource I wholeheartedly recommend for anyone embarking on the unique and beautiful journey of becoming a mother.

— Dr. Elliot Berlin, DC, founder of *Informed Pregnancy Media*

Introduction

Are you ready for one of your most life-changing experiences? We compare it to graduating from college, preparing for a promotion, or planning a wedding. Big life changes deserve attention. What you hold is the ultimate guide to help navigate this exciting and often overwhelming time of pregnancy, birth, and early parenting.

It doesn't matter if it is your first baby or third. It doesn't matter how you give birth. Every time you give birth, you become a mother all over again. Each pregnancy, birth, and baby is unique. There is no formula to follow, but we can help you understand your options and help you thrive.

The mission of our efforts here is to help reduce the anxiety and fear that comes along with pregnancy, birth, and parenting newborns.

We will guide and empower you so you know what questions to ask, how to plan, how to build your team to feel supported, and how to communicate your unique needs so you can confidently enter this new chapter of life excited and with all the tools you need to be prepared. With the right support, birth can be a transformative and empowering experience.

Our own experiences are what give us the drive to do this important work. We have not always been baby whisperers. Our births were not magical and without hurdles. I, Kristin, developed preeclampsia with my first and was induced at 39 weeks after some time on bedrest. My second birth was not without complications, I had postpartum hemorrhage after my son's quick, unmedicated birth.

Breastfeeding was not easy. In fact, I needed support from lactation consultants after both births. My first baby was in the NICU for four days due to glucose issues and relied on IV therapy, enhanced formula, and then my pumped milk. I needed help getting my daughter to latch. My second baby had a tongue tie and I struggled with mastitis. I had lactation consultants come to my home and visited the lactation consultants at the hospital. Alyssa and I both struggled with postpartum adjustments.

We want to give families information, resources, and expert advice that we wish we had while pregnant. We know that if we had a book like this, our postpartum experiences would have been quite different. We also would have felt more confident before giving birth.

We spent way too much time trying to research and prepare, and it would have been nice to have someone do the legwork for us as busy working professionals. That is why this book and the *Becoming A Mother* course exist. We didn't know how to ask for help when we needed it.

Do you?

Let us save you time and money as we give you support options and expert doula tips to better navigate pregnancy, birth, and early parenting.

Our book, *Supported*, is your one-stop-shop for everything you need to know about becoming a mother. It's written by two seasoned doulas with more than 19 years of combined experience who have helped more than 1,000 clients during pregnancy, birth, and early parenting.

The idea for *Supported* came out of a presentation we created in 2019 for a Bridal Expo about planning for birth and baby the way you would for a wedding. We wanted to reach couples early on to educate them about their support options. We loved the concept and carried that idea forward when we created the *Becoming A Mother* course during the early stages of the pandemic. Our clients were craving connection, so we decided to create a supportive community for mothers to engage with each other during a time when in-person classes were halted.

Most of *Part 1: Pregnancy and Birth Prep* in *Supported* is written by me, Kristin, and addresses the mindset and fears surrounding birth, providing resources to help build confidence as you prepare for birth and baby. We dive into assembling your dream team, and budgeting related to your unique needs. Jenni Froment, founder of VBAC Academy, shares tips on prepping for a vaginal birth after cesarean. We cover birth preparation, what classes to take, birth preferences, and top labor observations from an expert birth doula and certified birth coach. We have fitness and body balancing tips from Heidi McDowell of

Mind Body Baby GR. Dr. Angela Tallon, owner of Spirit Pediatrics covers newborn procedures in Chapter 5.

Part 2: Baby Prep and Setting Yourself Up for Postpartum Success is written by Alyssa and focuses on postpartum aspects of the experience, from parenting styles and communication to newborn care and sleep. It's everything we wish someone would have told us when we were pregnant! We have bonus sections on breastfeeding with advice from Kelly Emery, MSN, RN, IBCLC, and on postpartum mood and anxiety disorders from Cristina Stauffer, LMSW, as well as a list of our most trusted resources. Our former client, Lizzie Willams, offers some great tips for creating a baby registry with intention and thought.

Each chapter has personal stories from our former students and doula clients. We also have expert doula observations and tips. The birth prep section has some beautiful affirmations and meditations written by Amber Kilpatrick, spiritual ecologist and co-founder of Mindful School of Yoga™.

We want to help you have the most confident pregnancy, birth, and postpartum experience possible. Put your feet up and dive into this journey with us.

— Kristin Revere

Dedication

Brad, thank you for supporting me and believing in me through all of my wild ideas and new ventures. Finnley, you are my world. I love you both! I wouldn't be doing what I'm doing without either of you.

— Alyssa Veneklase

To the love of my life Patrick for eternally supporting me as a wife, mother, entrepreneur, and dreamer. I love you with all that I am. To Abbey and Seth who altered my life path from politics to birth work through my own unique pregnancy journeys with each of you. I love you both! To my bonus daughter Maddy for showing true determination and positivity through all of life's ups and downs. I love you. Thanks to my own family who formed who I am and for your support. To Anni Daulter who started me on the path to becoming a Sacred Pregnancy educator and then a doula. To Lori McCoy who taught me so much in my first doula training, I still view each birth as sacred. Thanks to my doulas, Chasity Moore and Juliea Paige who supported the birth of my son, Seth. To my Lamaze Instructor Diane Kutter, who always believed in my ability to have unmedicated births. Thanks to Kate Arnold and Chad Jones for asking me to be your travel birth and postpartum doula in Boston. I was honored to support you.

On the business side of things: shout out to Alex Batdorf, CEO of Get Sh!t Done for always setting me straight, many props go to the Nasdaq Milestone Circles team, Hey Mama connectors, and my mentors, Shenandoah Davis, and Nneka Hall. To Randy Patterson, CEO of ProDoula, for showing me that I could create a thriving doula agency. Many thanks to Tonya Sakowicz and the team at Newborn Care Solutions for your support and inspiration. Cheers to all the past and present team members of Gold Coast Doulas. You are all amazing. Much love to my doula agency owner besties: Andrea Stainbrook, Amy Hammer, Lindsey Thompson, Andrea Showers, and Shannon Barnett.

Thanks to Bianca Sprague, founder of Bebo Mia for being a fierce advocate for women.

Couldn't do it without the support and encouragement from my Zeta sisters. I so appreciate my dear friends Heather Zinn, Craig Stucky, Alicia and Michael Pavona, and Janette Glasco for bringing so much fun into my life. Thanks to my best friend Luisa Schumacher for always making me laugh and encouraging me to be bold. I can't forget all the moms who get things done and have watched my kids, sent photos from a field trip, or helped with sporting event transportation. It seriously takes a village, and we look out for each other.

Special thanks to Alyssa for dreaming big dreams with me on our various projects. You are the yin to my yang. Thanks to my current and former birth and postpartum doula clients who have allowed me into your lives and your birthing spaces, I carry you with me and dedicate this book to you.

— Kristin Revere

PART 1

Pregnancy and Birth Prep

CHAPTER 1

You're Pregnant! Now What?

For some women, pregnancy is welcomed news and for others it is unexpected or stressful. No matter what, this time is life-changing in many ways. We are here to help you navigate this season with resources and support.

Take a deep breath and let's get started.

Are you thinking positive thoughts or are they filled with fear? Our goal is to take the fear away and leave you feeling empowered.

Now is the time to think about your ideal birth. Start each day connecting with your baby and dreaming of the perfect birth for you. If you aren't familiar with visualization, we recommend *Visualizations for an Easier Childbirth* by Carl Jones and *HypnoBirthing: The Mongan Method* by Marie F. Mongan, M.ED., M.Hy. These resources are suggested for everything from unmedicated births to epidurals, to planned surgical births. I also love the *Mama Natural Pregnancy Cards* by Genevieve Howland. If you tend to be more logical and fact-based you could choose specific goals and think about how you are going to achieve them. I use some of these tools as a certified transformational birth coach.

Is there anything that worries you about childbirth? What might ease that worry?

During my second pregnancy, at the suggestion of my doulas and naturopath, I started each day with prayer, visualization, and deep yogic breathing. This sets the tone for the entire day. I had affirmations written out. I read aloud as I sipped on tea and visualized my birth. Many elite athletes use visualization to achieve their goals, and you can too. I ended each day the same way. It was a great way to carve out that time to focus on my birth and baby. I also tried to get a good sleep each night.

Do you feel connected to your baby? It is OK if you don't.

Some ways to connect involve singing, reading, or simply talking to your baby. If you have a partner, involve your partner as well. This helps them feel more bonded before your birth. If you have children, have them talk to the baby or babies while touching your growing belly. Some love to make art or pictures of their growing family. Allow them to share their dreams with their new sibling or siblings. Check out the book *Sacred Pregnancy* by Anni Daulter for tips on connection. It helped me so much with my second pregnancy as I faced the stress of potentially getting preeclampsia again.

Are you feeling connected to others during this time? If you have a partner, make time for date nights in or out. Walks are a great way to bond and talk about your dreams and goals. Build a strong community of others who support you and your dreams. People who are safe and will love and build you up positively as you navigate this season. Stay away from friends who want to tell you their horror stories about labor.

You may have fears during this time in your pregnancy. Some mothers fear labor, others fear becoming a mother for the first time or expanding the family. Some carry traumas from previous births, surgeries, or other experiences. Fear also could be acquired from the stories of others.

These feelings can be overwhelming, and it is great to talk to a therapist if possible. Childbirth classes like HypnoBirthing offer what is known as a fear release, which involves working through the fears and feelings to provide clarity on what can be worked through and let go.

Before we created the *Becoming A Mother* online course, we surveyed women in pregnancy groups about their fears: The most common were the fear of the unknown, pain, pooping during delivery, fear of giving birth on the way to the hospital, having an emergency cesarean, losing the baby, complications during labor, water breaking in public, failure to breastfeed, having a long labor, if my partner sees our baby get born will it change our relationship, dying during childbirth, getting postpartum depression, and not being a good mother. Some of these fears are heavy and others are a bit lighter in nature but can still be a big deal to the individual.

What is your biggest fear and how can you best prepare to overcome it?

If you have a partner, have you communicated your worries to them? You could also take this time to ask your partner about any fears they have. Working through the fears together creates a stronger connection and bond between couples in these transitions.

Body Image

It can be helpful to address your changing body and how you feel about the changes. I loved having curves for the first time and admired my belly as I passed storefront windows, but not everyone feels that way. Some of my former students expressed concern about weight gain during pregnancy or not being able to lose baby weight after.

Plus-size women may receive unwanted comments from friends, family members, or healthcare providers related to their size. If you fall into this category based on your body mass index, you may feel stressed about being labeled high-risk. I have supported many plus-size clients who had easy pregnancies and smooth births. They also had a supportive provider. I am a big fan of Jen McLellan of Plus Size Birth. Check out her website in our resources section and give a listen to her *Plus Mommy* podcast. She has an amazing pregnancy guide and a very comprehensive maternity guide. Jen recently trained our birth and postpartum team, so we can better empower and serve our clients.

If you have had an eating disorder, pregnancy can be an exceptionally difficult time and is best navigated with your healthcare team. Many clients have benefitted from adding a nutritionist or dietician to their team.

I tell my doula clients to focus on rest, hydration, and nourishing the body and baby during pregnancy. The American College of Obstetricians and Gynecologists recommends drinking eight to 12 glasses of water a day.

Put healthy food in your body. What are your cravings? Are you intentional about what you eat? I am a big fan of the book *Real Food for Pregnancy* by Lily Nichols, RDN, CDE, as a great source of nutrition information. She also wrote *Real Food for Gestational Diabetes*; I refer to that book often as well.

I recently interviewed Katie Timbrook, the chief nutrition officer at Athena's Bump on *Ask the Doulas* and learned that they offer free customized recipes based on unique needs during pregnancy, as well as for meals in the fourth trimester. I would have loved this option when I was pregnant and post-delivery.

Make it a priority to rest. Rest helps your body replenish itself and is shown to reduce stress and improve mood.

Self-Care

Self-care is the buzzword everywhere you look, but in my opinion, the advice is shallow and often is focused on being pampered, like getting a pedicure or facial. Don't get me wrong, those things are great, and self-care can be different for every person, but during pregnancy the focus may be better placed on less cosmetic but more mind and body support. Think about what relaxes you and incorporate that into your self-care routine.

What does that self-care look like for you?

Here are some tips from our clients and students from surveys we put out in mom groups before creating the *Becoming A Mother* course launched:

"Get out and do things during pregnancy while you have the freedom."

"Learn to take steps forward and don't try to make your old life and expectations fit into your new life."

"Embrace the necessity to slow down."

"Stop cleaning so much."

"Move your body everyday if you are physically able."

"Pinterest and Instagram are fake. Stop trying to compete with curated versions of pregnancy and parenting."

"Avoid Google, it will only scare you."

"Women in pregnancy and mom groups often aren't experts, you don't need to listen to their advice."

Remember, you are unique and so is your individual birth and parenting journey. This is not your mother's birth, your sister's, or your friend's, it is your pregnancy and birth now, and you don't get a do-over.

PREGNANCY PREP STORY

🗩 Lindsay Carlson, former doula client

"The day before my labor started was a difficult one emotionally. I was ready to have my baby. My husband suggested that maybe the emotions were a sign labor was close. To take care of myself that night, I took a bath and, in the bath, I did a visualization of the birth. I thought about what I liked about my previous births (labor building into the evening), and what I didn't like (laboring the entire night and into the next morning). So, I pictured laboring at home and driving to the hospital. I thought about how dilated I wanted to be when we arrived. I thought about what it would feel like when I got to the birthing room and how long I would labor there, when my waters would release, and in what position I would want to push. It was a peaceful preparation that helped me align my mind with my body."

📢 An affirmation from spiritual ecologist Amber Kilpatrick

"I give myself permission to feel happy, sad, worried, excited, ready, not ready, hopeful, and everything in between. Motherhood is vast. Feeling into that vastness requires many emotions."

📋 Doula Observation from Kristin

Surround yourself with positive people and stories. Birth is as mental as it is physical. Prep for birth the way you would prep for an athletic event that involves both mind and body. Check out our "Ask the Doulas" podcast episode on the topic at the following address: www.goldcoastdoulas.com/train-for-birth-the-way-you-would-for-an-ironman-podcast-episide-234/

CHAPTER 2

Assembling Your Dream Team of Personal and Professional Support

Couples spend time and money hiring planners and invest in their dream wedding, but childbirth is often an overlooked, though much-needed, life event where professional support plays a large role. The average wedding[1] costs $30,000 in 2022 according to *The Knot*. This was a $2,000 increase from 2021. Couples often spend a year or more planning for a wedding, but often feel that birth and postpartum planning will take care of itself.

With that in mind, here are some of my tips as an expert doula on how to build your dream team.

Set time aside to discuss goals for your pregnancy, birth, and the newborn phase. Make a list and then narrow down what is most important to you.

You may value the emotional support and coaching from a doula throughout your pregnancy and during your birth. It can be reassuring to know that someone is there with you every step of the way. Others may value photo documentation during pregnancy, and of the new baby from a maternity and birth photographer. Some expenses like a doula or a childbirth class may be covered under an HSA or FSA account. Other expenses, such as a breast pump, can qualify for insurance coverage.

You also have some self-paid expenses to budget, such as photography or videography.

Once you decide on a budget, you can map out when payments are due. Many birth and baby professionals accept payment plans. Some of these include maternity photographers, videographers, birth doulas, postpartum and infant care doulas. We will get into their definitions in just a bit.

Add services versus "things" to your baby shower and sprinkles. Check out the online registry, Be Her Village, that is focused on giving you cash for the services and support you need.

Are you overwhelmed at the thought of bringing your baby home when you know your partner has to go back to work right away? Babies don't come with instruction manuals, and you likely will be exhausted after giving birth. Imagine if someone could not only be there to support you but is also an expert in newborn care. They can make sure you are drinking water and bring you healthy snacks. They can vacuum your living room as you know you shouldn't be lifting after having a baby. They will help with feeding, spend time with an older child, and make sure you get needed rest as you heal. These are just some of the ways a postpartum and infant care doula can help.

Other great gifted items to consider are house cleaners, a diaper service, meal delivery service, and laundry service. Anything to make your life easier will be much appreciated and think of all the items you will keep out of the landfill. You really didn't need that eight pack of pink onesies anyway.

You don't have to do this alone!

We aren't made to be isolated after giving birth. Consider a mix of personal and professional support as you plan for this life transition the way you would plan for a wedding.

Let's dive into your personal and professional support team.

Your birth is an intimate and important time, and it is wise to carefully consider who you invite into that space. We will talk about who to bring onto your team and how you will pay for each professional.

Where Should I Give Birth?

If you are low risk, you should plan to give birth where you feel comfortable. Some people are more comfortable giving birth at home than in the hospital. Others want the security of the hospital. Some individuals are high-risk and need to deliver in a hospital.

Hospital

In the United States, 98.4 percent of people give birth in the hospital.[2] Most often there will be multiple hospitals in your area to choose from, usually with an array of birthing options. For example, a hospital in my area offers natural birthing suites for low-risk patients as an alternative to a regular hospital room. They look more like a hotel room and are often supported by nurse midwives. For high-risk individuals, it is of utmost importance to look at the level of neonatal intensive care when selecting a hospital. An example of this is if you are expecting twins or triplets.

Birth Centers

You can find birth centers attached to a hospital, or as freestanding organizations. Birth centers typically are supported by Certified Nurse Midwives (CNMs) or Certified Professional Midwives (CPMs) and can be a safe place for low-risk women to give birth. Nurse Midwives are sometimes overseen by an OB and freestanding birth centers often have transfer policies worked out with an area hospital. Insurance may cover birth center births, especially if they are connected to a hospital.

Your Home

Home birth is another option to consider for low-risk individuals. It is convenient as you don't need to travel during labor, and you have all of the comforts of home. In states where home birth is legal, you may be able to choose from a CPM or a CNM. Some states that aren't regulated also include traditional or lay midwives as an option.

When choosing your location, it is important to consider where you feel safe and who you want your medical team to consist of.

Sometimes your birthing location is dependent on who you choose to support you. Your provider may have hospital privileges at one or multiple hospitals.

Common Provider Options

Midwives

The term midwife means "with women". They often work with low-risk patients. There are many different types of midwives; here are the most common.

Certified Nurse Midwife (CNM)

Certified Nurse Midwives can attend births in hospitals, birth centers, and at home. However, not all CNMs attend home births. Nurse Midwives typically support low-risk patients. CNMs are educated in graduate-level midwifery programs accredited by ACME, according to the American College of Nurse Midwives. CNMs have an active RN credential at the time of the board certification exam. Many of them were former labor and delivery nurses.[3]

Certified Midwife (CM)

CMs have a bachelor's degree or higher in a health field or have completed an accredited midwifery education program and have passed a national exam. They are not required to be nurses but have similar training to a Certified Nurse Midwife.[4]

Certified Professional Midwife (CPM)

They are midwives who have clinical experience in childbirth and are also trained outside the hospital and have passed a national exam. Some CPMs hold an associate or bachelor's degree in direct-entry midwifery (DEM). CPMs mainly attend home births. There are also traditional midwives and lay midwives in some states. Some home birth midwives operate in a solo practice model with backup and others have partnerships or a team that may include birth assistants and apprentices. It is important to figure out what model of care makes the most sense for you.[4]

Physicians

There are multiple physician options depending on the location of the hospital you choose, including:

Obstetrician (OB)

These doctors specialize in obstetrics. They mainly work in hospitals and focus on pregnancy and delivering babies and many offer gynecological care (OB/GYN). They work with all types of pregnancies from low to high-risk and perform surgeries.

Family Practice Physician

These doctors care for entire families and sometimes attend labor and deliveries. They usually work with low-risk pregnancies, but some also offer high-risk support. A family practice doctor can replace a pediatrician.

Doctor of Osteopathic Medicine (DO)

DOs are licensed physicians who "emphasize a whole-person approach to treatment and care" according to the American Osteopathic Association (AOA).[5]

Maternal Fetal Medicine (MFM)

MFM Doctors work with high-risk patients and their babies. Some patients continue to see their OB in tandem with occasional MFM appointments.

Pediatrician

These doctors specialize in infants, children, and young adults. You also will want to choose your pediatrician during pregnancy as you will get asked who your pediatrician is during labor. You will want to check with your insurance company to make sure that pediatrician is "in network", if you will, and also ensure that the pediatrician is accepting new patients.

Choosing your Provider

Look at your goals for your birth and make sure your provider supports those goals. Some insurance plans limit provider options and hospital choices. Get recommendations from friends and health care professionals. Interview different providers. Do they make you feel comfortable and supported versus just tolerated? Does your provider take time to listen to your concerns? Are you comfortable asking sensitive questions? Does your provider share call in a practice model? Does their practice align with your birth preferences? Your OB may be amazing, but what if they aren't the doctor attending your birth? Can you meet other doctors or midwives in the practice during your prenatal visits?

How to Pay

Take a look at your insurance and see what provider and hospital options you have. Sometimes home birth midwives have prenatal visit insurance coverage where the birth is self-pay. You may need to self-pay for all of your home birth. Many times, the self-pay amount works out to be what a co-pay would be for a hospital birth. You may also be able to use a health savings account, health reimbursement arrangement, or flex spending account to pay for midwifery or additional hospital fees. Not all medical practices accept Medicaid, so that may also be a factor in choosing your provider. Your insurance should cover a portion or the majority of the hospital fees. Look into your coverage during pregnancy so you can figure out your budget and plan from there. When choosing your provider, it is also important to consider how supportive they are of your preferred birthing option.

Birthing Options

Vaginal Birth

Vaginal birth is the most common method of childbirth. The birthing person delivers their baby or babies through the vagina. This could be medicated or unmedicated.

Unmedicated

The birthing person relies on their own hormones to help labor progress. They can move around throughout labor. One of the benefits is the lack of side effects to the birthing person and baby. They may experience a shorter labor and shorter pushing phase when compared to women who give birth with an epidural.[6]

Medicated

Medicated birth is the most common type of vaginal delivery in the United States. More than 73 percent of hospital births in 2015 used epidurals or spinal blocks for pain relief.[7]

MEDICAL PAIN RELIEF FOR BIRTH INCLUDE THE FOLLOWING

IV Pain Meds

IV pain meds can help to take the edge off labor and help calm the birthing person. They are known as opioids. They can make you and/or your baby feel drowsy or loopy. Some examples are Demerol, Stadol, and Nubain.

Nitrous Oxide

Also known as laughing gas, nitrous oxide will take the edge off without affecting the baby. It does not eliminate pain completely. It is a lower dosage than you would get at the dentist's office.

Epidural Anesthesia

Epidural Anesthesia is the most common form of labor pain relief. It can be helpful to allow rest and reduce pain. It is an injection of local anesthetic in the space around the spinal nerves in the lower back to block pain from contractions. They can be done during any stage of labor but are most common in the first stage. Cons: may decrease blood pressure, may slow baby's heart rate.[8]

Cesarean Birth

A cesarean may be planned elective or an unplanned surgical birth. Some birthing persons with medical complications may be a favorable candidate for a cesarean delivery. Recovery often is longer than that for a vaginal birth. Risks include blood loss and blood clots, among other potential complications from the surgery that include a higher maternal mortality, higher risk of complications in future pregnancies, a higher likelihood of infant breathing issues, as well as NICU stays.

Family Centered Cesarean/Gentle Cesareans

As a doula, I have supported many family-centered cesareans, also known as gentle cesareans. It can be beneficial to discuss options for a gentle cesarean with your provider and come up with a plan. Options may include clear drapes with a pass-through flap, playing music at the birth, delayed cord clamping, immediate skin-to-skin, or immediate breastfeeding. If you have one, ask if your doula can be in the room. A hospital in my area even has a camera system where you can watch the entire process or just look at the screen when your baby is born.

Vaginal Birth After Cesarean/Trial of Labor after Cesarean

I asked Jenni Froment to contribute to this section on VBAC/TOLAC. She is the founder of VBAC Academy and is a certified birth doula. I am certified through VBAC Academy and know that Jenni is such a great resource for doulas and parents alike on VBACs.

Planning a VBAC can feel like a full-time job, and I remember feeling like the mental weight of all the planning really sucked the joy out of my pregnancy. That's why in 2015 I started a journey to make it easier for VBAC parents to plan and achieve VBAC births. In 2017, I expanded to include training local doulas on how to better support and educate their VBAC clients. In 2020, I launched VBAC Academy to make planning a VBAC easier for people across the world.

VBAC often feels like a radical act of rebellion in the birth world, with many birth providers in the U.S. and around the world still actively enforcing VBAC rules that are outdated, and not based on research or evidence.

In 2010, the American College of Ob-Gyn (ACOG) officially declared VBAC the safe and reasonable choice for women with one or two previous cesareans, who would otherwise be a candidate for VBAC.

The good news is all that planning pays off and VBAC birthers can boast a successful VBAC rate of up to 80 percent in many research studies. In fact, VBAC birthers have cesarean rates as low as 20 percent compared to most national averages of about 30 percent.

Said another way, VBAC planners are really good at avoiding cesareans because we pour over research, scour the internet, follow all the VBAC sites, and learn how to make our own choices in the absence of a birth system that's supportive enough or well-enough informed on VBAC births. We often spend our entire pregnancies feeling like we are fighting against the system, and constantly having to defend our right to make choices about our pregnancy or delivery.

It's been eight years since I had my second VBA2C (vaginal birth after two cesareans) birth, and I am still faced with looks of shock and horror when I mention that I had a vaginal birth after two cesareans. Those looks only serve to remind me that the people planning VBACs today are still dealing with that nonsense, and I have work to do.

If you are pregnant and planning a VBAC, there are five key steps I recommend to maximize your experience and simplify your efforts so you can enjoy your pregnancy and birth experience, even if things change and you need a cesarean.

1. Choose a supportive VBAC provider

First, picking your VBAC dream team is invaluable. Choosing a doula that has specialized VBAC certification in their skillset will take a considerable mental load from you. Importantly, they can also assist you in selecting a truly supporting VBAC birth provider. Midwives and Obstetricians are the most common birth providers for VBAC, but there are hundreds of variations of birth providers and rules that vary by location that change who can support which types. Having a doula with you to sort through your options and prepare you for the questions to ask can save valuable time.

2. Review interventions carefully

Remember that interventions can save or sabotage your chances for a vaginal birth, depending on the scenario. We can have the position that we want to avoid interventions, but sometimes they can help us achieve the vaginal birth we are striving for. Most people would choose Pitocin over a repeat cesarean if they needed to progress labor; and sometimes epidurals can give someone the rest they need to push a baby out after a long and difficult labor. It's easy to slip into a black and white mindset when birth planning because avoiding a cesarean feels so important, but it's important to accept that sometimes the plan changes and giving yourself permission to change your mind can offer significant mental peace before and during labor. When presented with an intervention during pregnancy or labor, the goal is to understand what the test or procedure is, why the provider thinks it's necessary, what the alternative options are and what the included risks are of the intervention. With that full view of the situation, you'll feel more confident in your decision making. This step specifically supports the high success rate of VBAC birthers because we avoid interventions that increase our chances of a repeat cesarean unnecessarily but know when to use interventions to help us get to the vaginal birth finish line.

3. Do your birth planning and know your birth rights

The third step in planning a VBAC birth is understanding that making your birth plan is an exercise in educating yourself, not a recipe or precise roadmap for getting from pregnant to un-pregnant. There is no way to prepare for every single possible birth variable, so the better method is to prepare for dealing with the unknown. I do not typically recommend hospital birth classes; they are motivated to teach you based on what their policies are versus what is physiologically normal. I also recommend taking both a birth class and a VBAC class or hiring a VBAC PRO doula to support you in birth planning. There are VBAC-specific birth classes available at VBAC Academy, that can offer you specialized VBAC information and advice to supplement your birth planning. I highly recommend making a plan for how to approach choices in pregnancy or delivery so that you can feel informed and confident in your decision making. A big influencing factor in feeling "good" after birth is feeling respected and "in-control" of your body and birth during the process. Having a plan for the unexpected will help you feel more prepared and can avoid stressful labor situations.

4. Prepare your whole self for birth; deal with your fears

The fourth step of VBAC planning reminds us to prepare our whole self for labor. Simply said, if you spend your whole pregnancy planning for the birth but neglect to plan for how to cope when birth gets hard and you want to quit? You're doing yourself a tremendous disservice. It's true that VBAC birthers go into birth with a lot more expectations and mental baggage than those not birthing after cesarean. We have all kinds of triggers that can trip us up during childbirth. As a self-identified Type-A, control-freak, I struggled to let go of expectations in my first VBA2C and I regretted the feeling that I survived a battle after my birth instead of feeling empowered and appreciative of my body. For my second birth, I focused entirely on what I needed to do to enjoy my birth experience and how I could build trust in my mind and body so that I didn't need to manage this process. I had everything I needed inside of me. I just had to let my body do its thing. Teaching pregnant people how to achieve this level of preparedness has been an important piece of my VBAC message since I opened my birth business. Yes, we want to VBAC and we have a lot of planning to do, but also this is your baby's only birth and I want you to try to enjoy this story as it unfolds. Ask yourself what you need to do to process your fears about birth before you enter the birth space so that you can be present, and maybe even joyful.

5. Prepare for a Gentle Cesarean Birth (just in case)

No one likes to plan for a cesarean when they are planning for a VBAC but I'll tell you what's worse: needing a cesarean, after planning for a VBAC—and not having a plan. There is a type of cesarean protocol called a "Gentle Cesarean"; it's practiced across the United States and across the world but access to the protocol varies greatly by local areas. The term refers to a collection of birth choices available during a cesarean birth that traditionally have not been included. The options include delayed cord clamping, skin-to-skin in the OR, and clear drapes so that parents can easily watch their baby being born.

Those details can make a big difference in feeling present and a part of your birth experience. Also, it's OK to be disappointed in your birth experience and grateful that everything is OK. This is part of the emotional work to focus on while planning for your VBAC.

Planning a VBAC is hard work, but there have been trailblazers paving the way to help make this easier. Reading this book is a great start for building a strong foundation in planning an optimal birth and postpartum experience, and next you'll need a couple of supplemental resources to help prepare you for your unique VBAC journey. Those can be found in the resources section at the back of the book.

— Jenni Froment

Inductions

Again, this book is not a childbirth education manual, so I will only touch on this topic. There are many types of inductions, ranging from using cervical ripeners to synthetic oxytocin under the brand name Pitocin. My favorite resource for induction information is *Evidence-Based Birth*. Check out the article on *Inducing for Due Dates*[9], the article on *Big Babies*[10] and the *Pocket Guide to Interventions*.

Birth Doula Support

What is a birth doula anyway?

Birth doulas provide non-judgmental, non-medical support to the clients and families during labor, birth, and immediately after delivery. Doulas know about birth; your partner knows you and your provider takes care of you and your baby, which makes for a great team.

Should you hire a doula?

My vote is yes after having doula support at my second birth and no support with my first. Labor can be an intense physical, emotional, and exhausting experience.

My husband was cautious about hiring doulas for our second birth as he didn't want to feel replaced. After we hired our team he said it was the best decision, as he could support me emotionally and not worry about anything else. With our first birth, he kept referring to our Lamaze manual when interventions were suggested. Partners are sometimes cautious about doulas at first and they can end up being our biggest fans afterward.

Some women want that emotional support or coaching during labor. It can be helpful to have physical touch like hip squeezes and counter-pressure, or assistance with moving and changing positions in labor. You may want informational support or guidance in creating a birth plan. Doulas can give encouragement and help you communicate your wishes to your medical team. Your doula can show your partner how to support you and offer them time to go eat or take a break knowing you have constant support.

Doulas can support all types of birth from home to hospital, medicated to unmedicated, and vaginal to surgical. Many people only associate doulas with home births or unmedicated births. Doulas also work as a team with nurses and doctors or midwives. You may have an amazing nurse, but they are responsible for charting and monitoring you and baby or babies. You may end up with more than one nurse depending on shift changes. Doulas know you well from connecting with you during pregnancy, and they understand how you want to be supported.

How Do Doulas Practice?

Not all doulas are the same. Some prefer to attend only home births and others attend all types of births including surgical and epidurals. Doulas aren't regulated, so if certification is important to you, then it's important to ask questions about training and certification status. Some doulas work in a team or with an agency and have a shared call method of care. With the shared call method, two doulas support you in pregnancy and one attends your birth. Other doulas work in a larger practice and have on-call days the way physicians do. Some doulas work alone and rely on backups in case of illness or emergency.

How To Find a Birth or Postpartum Doula

There are so many ways to find a good doula. You can ask your provider for recommendations or ask friends who have benefited from doula support.

It is important to look at both personality and experience when hiring a doula for birth or postpartum and infant care. You can find doulas through sites like DoulaMatch.com by typing in your zip code and due date. Another option is to Google "doulas near me". Always look for documentation on a doula's credentials as well as client reviews. Many hospitals only allowed certified doulas in during the COVID pandemic, for example. Most insurance plans like Carrot Fertility require certified and insured doulas.

Some doulas offer free consultations. It is helpful to ask about their philosophy and style to make sure that you have found the perfect fit. The doulas at Gold Coast tell our clients about our superpowers, like the ability to read a room and anticipate needs before a client or partner asks for support.

Questions for Doulas

Here are some questions you might ask a potential doula during the interview:

- What is your backup plan?
- When do you begin your call time?
- How many births have you attended?
- What is your experience related to birth support? For example, do you have experience with supporting high risk clients or twin births?
- What is your biggest strength as a member of my birth team?
- How will you support my partner?
- What does your support during my pregnancy look like?
- How long do you stay after delivery?
- When do you arrive at the birth?
- Do you have an hourly rate after a certain amount of in-person labor support?
- Do you offer a follow-up postpartum visit?

It is important for you to connect personally with your doula as well as feel confident about their experience. I am one who goes on instinct. I hired my doulas based on the gut feeling after the interview. I did not interview other options but may have if the connection wasn't there. Other mothers have a list of questions and are more analytical in nature. Some feel like they connected well with the doula and that they would be friends. Do what is best for your personality and expectations. If you have a partner, it is also helpful to get them on board and include them in the selection process.

Evidence in Support of Doulas

"We have long known the threat of maternal mortality and morbidity is especially acute for women of color. The rate of maternal deaths among Black women nearly doubled and rates for Hispanic women more than doubled from 2019 to 2021. The fact remains that the U.S. healthcare system has historically failed people of color, including during the crucial times of pregnancy and postpartum."

— Dr. Elizabeth Cherot, March of Dimes
Senior Vice President and Chief Medical Officer

Maternal Health and Mortality

The statistics are scary, but the topic of maternal health and mortality are too important to gloss over. We added this section to illustrate how effective doula support and care can be at preventing unnecessary negative outcomes. Doula support should be considered an essential part of every person's pregnancy, labor, and postpartum experience. We will go into more detail about statistics shortly.

According to the Centers for Disease Control and Prevention, approximately 700 women die each year in the United States as a result of pregnancy or delivery complications. Almost two-thirds of pregnancy-related deaths are preventable.

In 2020, Black women were most disproportionately affected, with a mortality rate of 55.3 deaths per 100,000 live births, compared to 19.1 deaths, and 18.2 deaths per 100,000 live births for white and Hispanic women, respectively, according to the CDC.

In 2020, the maternal mortality rate for Black women was three times the rate for white women in the United States. Multiple factors contribute to these disparities, such as lower quality healthcare, structural racism, implicit bias from healthcare providers, and underlying chronic conditions.

The U.S. has an infant mortality rate of 5.4 per 1,000 live births with a health disparity among Black babies[11] at a rate of 10.6 deaths per 1,000 live births.

Don't be fooled, these statistics for Black women are not only for low-income women. You may have heard Serena William's story or watched her documentary. It is a prime example that all Black women are affected and face bias within the healthcare system, regardless of education, income level, or any other demographic.

We are thankful for organizations like Hello Seven Foundation, which provides vouchers for birth and postpartum doulas to help black birthing people in need.

Alyssa and I have been working on advocating for doulas to be added to insurance for years. We worked closely with our consultant, Katherine Steffy, to collect data. This research can be found in the external references section at the back of the book under Maternal Health and Mortality.

Here is some of what we learned together through years of advocating for doulas and insurance:

Knowing the crucial role doulas play in long-term outcomes for both mother and baby, we think it's a no-brainer for doulas to be covered as a necessity of birth. From an equity lens, doulas should be essential. Black, American Indians, and Pacific Islanders are at a greater risk than white Americans to have preterm births, low birth-weight babies, or receive late or no prenatal care. Hispanic women are twice as likely as white women to receive late or no prenatal care.

There were 12 separate randomized trials that compared outcomes between labors supported by doulas and those that were not. They found that doula support significantly reduced the length of labor and the odds of medical interventions including cesarean section, forceps delivery, Pitocin, and pharmaceutical pain relief. Doulas were also known to reduce anxiety levels and increase satisfaction with the birth regardless of the outcome. Evaluations of partner-only or other non-doula support did not see the same results.[12]

The impact doulas have on quality of care and clinical outcomes cannot be overstated because their work ultimately affects not just one client, but two or more. Doulas empower mothers to fully participate in their care decisions.

Doulas work as a team with healthcare providers to...

- Facilitate communication and decision-making with the clinical care team
- Allow nurses to refocus from emotional needs to clinical ones
- Improve birth satisfaction, regardless of delivery type
- Can alleviate quality, cost, and satisfaction issues related to pregnancy and birth

Doulas Are...

- Supported by the American College of Obstetricians and Gynecologists
- Supported by the Society for Maternal-Fetal Medicine

Moms with doula support...

- Experience shorter labors
- Are 40 percent less likely to need a cesarean section
- Are less likely to require an instrumental birth or regional analgesia
- Are less likely to use Pitocin, which has been linked to NICU utilization
- Are more likely to be satisfied with their birth regardless of outcomes.
- Are more likely to initiate and sustain breastfeeding, providing health benefits for both mom and baby, ranging from reduced postpartum bleeding to reduced cancer risks for mom to reduced diabetes risks for babies

Babies born with doula support are...

- Four times less likely to be low birth weight
- 25 percent less likely to be pre-term
- Less likely to have low 1- and 5-minute Apgar scores
- More likely to breastfeed, and for a longer duration

Pre-term birth and low birthweight are leading causes for infant mortality. Having appropriate prenatal and birth support can help babies avoid the factors that negatively impact their health. Birth doulas play an important role in this support.

Working with Katherine Steffy over the last ten years on insurance for doulas led us to believe that good data in this space is relatively new and has been difficult to come by. There is potentially some selection bias happening as the individuals who currently have doulas or would have had doulas for these studies tend to be self-pay and may already have been in the position to better access resources, be health literate, be actively participating in care decisions, and ultimately may have had better outcomes anyway. As a result, the benefits of doulas often go unrecognized, because we aren't getting doula care to the patients who could most benefit from it. Self-funded insurance programs and state Medicaid programs are important in making equitable change.

Other Types of Doulas

Fertility Doulas

Fertility doulas offer emotional and informational support during the conception process. Some offer education and many assist in understanding your options.

Bereavement (Loss) Doulas

Loss doulas support miscarriage, stillbirth, and infant loss. They can support families with known loss during the entire pregnancy and birth or offer support and resources after a loss.

Antepartum Doulas

If you are high-risk, you can also work with an antepartum or bed rest doula to help with emotional support, meal preparation, childbirth prep, nursery setup, and household tasks. They can provide sibling care if you have other children. Antepartum doulas support clients at home and in the hospital. Some conditions that can benefit from a bed rest doula are preeclampsia, carrying multiples, previous complications, placenta previa, and premature labor. Bed rest may be strict, restricted, or modified, I was on modified bed rest when I had preeclampsia with my first pregnancy. I could get up a few times a day.

Postpartum Doulas and Newborn Care Specialists (NCS)

You may want to consider day or overnight postpartum care during your healing phase. Postpartum doulas can help with the newborn in hospital or home after delivery. Many doulas and NCS work for the first few months and some postpartum doulas work through the first year. What is the difference between a postpartum doula and a newborn care specialist? A newborn care specialist (NCS) is trained to care for the newborn while postpartum doulas focus on caring for the entire family including the newborn and mother during recovery. NCS tend to offer live-in, travel and 24-7 support. Doulas also do household tasks where a NCS does not. They are both wonderful options. Some postpartum doulas are also newborn care specialists. Doulas and NCS can support all types of feeding.

Moola for the Doula

Once you decide on your budget it is time to interview your dream team.

It is important to look at both personality and experience when hiring a doula for birth or postpartum care as I mentioned earlier when discussing birth doulas.

Some states have Medicaid coverage for birth doulas. Our own home state of Michigan just added Medicaid for doulas in January 2023, yay! General insurance does not currently cover doulas, but more companies are beginning to add birth and postpartum doula services to their maternity benefits.

Gold Coast Doulas was featured in an article in *The Washington Post* publication, *The Lily*, that profiled companies like CVS and

Microsoft for adding doulas to benefit packages. Our partnership with a local company, Pioneer Construction, made the story as well. Pioneer Construction added both birth and postpartum doula support to their benefits plan. Since then, Amazon, Hearst Communications, LinkedIn, PNC Bank, Salesforce, Walmart, and Target have added doula support to their benefits packages. I can't wait to see who else comes on board. Some companies offer benefits through Carrot Fertility or Progyny. TRICARE military insurance covers doulas under certain plans. Some doulas offer a military discount if they don't accept TRICARE.

You can make changes by speaking to your employer about adding doulas to their benefits package. For information on navigating your family benefits, check out The Park Consulting. I learned so much about parental leave from my interview with Linzay Davis on *Ask the Doulas* podcast.

There are also some healthcare sharing programs that pay part of the fee for doula support. Those include Samaritan Ministries and Christian Healthcare Ministries.

Your HSA or FSA may cover postpartum doula support in addition to birth doulas. If not, set up a registry on Be Her Village to get funds to pay for doulas, childbirth education, lactation, and more. Most doulas are self-pay and offer payment plans. There are some grant-funded, community-based doula plans, and pro-bono hospital-based doula programs. You may also find some nonprofits to help with volunteers in the home after baby arrives. An example of this is MomsBloom, in West Michigan.

Other birth and prenatal team members

We like to say if you don't know your options for support, you have none. You may want to consider adding some of these members to your prenatal and birth dream team and work out a budget the way you would for a wedding. I am including my favorites, but there are certainly many others that I haven't listed.

Birth Photographer

Birth photographers are on call for your birth the way a doula is. They capture the labor, delivery, and the hour following birth. They attend births in home, hospital, and birth centers. They often provide maternity and newborn photography. Some offer videography services, as well. This is a self-pay service.

Cord Blood Banking or Donation

Consider cord blood donation or cord blood banking. Cord Blood Banking is when your baby's umbilical cord blood is collected and stored after delivery. If you donate to a public bank, families can look to a bank for donors to try to find a match for their child. We did a podcast years ago with Anja Health and the founder Kathryn Cross told us that cord blood has been FDA approved to treat sickle cell anemia and diabetes. Either way, you get a collection kit in advance of your birth, and you bring it to the hospital or give it to your home birth midwife. For banking, you would fill out a form and ship off the kit after collection. Donation kits can be mailed or dropped off if there are local donation sites. Some hospitals partner with donation sites and collect and return kits onsite. For more information about cord blood banking check out www.anjahealth.com or www.viacord.com. For info on donating cord blood, check out www.bethematch.org.

Baby Registry Expert

Baby registry consultants help families build their gift registries for both products as well as services. They are baby gear experts that customize support based on each client's unique needs. You can find certified gift registry experts at Babylist, Be Her Village or by searching Google. Services are often virtual as well as in-person. We recently added this service for our clients, and it is well received.

Placenta Encapsulation

Placenta encapsulators are on call for a birth, as well, and pick up the placenta after delivery. Some doulas are also encapsulators. The placenta is steamed, dehydrated, and crushed into capsules. Some encapsulators also make tinctures or raw smoothies. There are two main methods of encapsulation: raw and traditional Chinese method (TCM). This is not a regulated industry. Anecdotally, their consumption shows evidence of increased milk supply and decreased risk of postpartum depression. This is a self-pay service.[13]

Many of the services below are covered by insurance or HSA/FSA accounts, depending on the provider's payment options

Webster Certified Chiropractor

These chiropractic doctors have specialized in the care of prenatal patients. The Webster Method aligns the pelvis and includes a soft tissue release of associated muscle groups. This method can be great for positioning and relieving discomfort.

Physical Therapist

Seeing a physical therapist can relieve the aches and pains of pregnancy. I often recommend that my clients see a physical therapist. They can also give their patients stretches and exercises to do at home.

Pelvic Floor Therapist

Pelvic floor physical therapy is a specialty area within physical therapy focusing on the rehabilitation of muscles in the pelvic floor. This can be helpful during pregnancy and in the postnatal phase. We will talk about the benefits of pelvic floor therapy later in the book when we address postpartum recovery. www.webmd.com/women/what-is-pelvic-floor-physical-therapy.

Prenatal Massage Therapist

Massages are performed by a licensed prenatal massage therapist and are tailored to the needs of pregnant women and their changing bodies. Some prenatal massage therapists have tables with cut outs to help make pregnant women more comfortable.

Mental Health Therapist

There are many types of mental health professionals including Licensed Clinical Social Workers (LMSW), Licensed Professional Counselors (LPC), LMFT, Licensed Marriage and Family Therapists, Psychiatrists, and Psychologists. Some therapists specialize in perinatal mood disorders (PMADs), which will be covered in chapters to come. Sessions are either virtual or in-person depending on the provider.

Acupuncturist

Acupuncture involves the insertion of very fine needles through the skin at strategic points in your body. A key component of traditional Chinese medicine (TCM), acupuncture is most commonly used to treat pain. Increasingly, it is being used for overall wellness, including stress management. Acupuncture can be helpful in so many ways during pregnancy such as inducing labor, flipping a breech baby, reducing anxiety, and nausea. Many acupuncturists also offer acupressure, which is a similar method administered with pressure rather than a needle.

Functional Medicine Doctor

According to The Cleveland Clinic[14], functional medicine uses a holistic approach to treat chronic disease, with a focus on nutrition. I often send clients to a functional medicine provider if they have conditions like gestational diabetes, hyperemesis gravidarum (HG), thyroid disorders, or food allergies.

Doctor of Naturopathic Medicine (ND)

They are educated and trained in accredited naturopathic medical colleges. An ND can create individualized health plans for mothers during pregnancy and in the postnatal phase. They care for the whole person.[15]

Nutritionist

Nutritionists can help with diet, allergies, health problems, and they can formulate special menus for clients. Licensing varies from state to state. A nutritionist tends to be more generalized where dieticians work in specialized areas. This may or may not be covered by insurance.[16]

Dietician (RD or RDN)

They are certified to treat clinical conditions. They tend to work in specialized areas and monitor or address concerns and offer viable solutions to problems. This often is covered by insurance.[17]

Craniosacral Therapist (CST)

This type of practitioner uses a gentle hands-on technique with light touch to examine membranes and movements of the fluids in and around the central nervous system.[18] It can be helpful during pregnancy and postnatal recovery. Newborns can also benefit from CST. I often refer clients to a craniosacral therapist if there are feeding challenges with a baby.

Other newborn services to consider budgeting for are baby sign language classes, music classes, and infant massage.

Partner and Family Support

Have you truly thought about who you want to attend your birth? Would you rather it just be you and your partner, or do you want family members and friends to attend as well? Visitor policies vary at each hospital. Understand that no matter where or how you choose to give birth, your personal support team should enhance your birth rather than cause more tension and stress. You don't get a do-over on this birth. Have the difficult decisions about who you want to attend your birth earlier in pregnancy rather than waiting until you go into labor.

Some clients also choose to wait until they get home to have visitors to focus on rest and bonding. That is also a personal decision that should be communicated early with family and friends. Do you want to rely on family to watch your pets or other kids? This should also be communicated early on.

If you have a tight budget, ask for help from family and friends.

Your friends and family want to help, but they aren't mind readers. If your friends haven't had babies themselves, they may think that you want to be left alone. Many times, taking care of a newborn can be isolating. What friends could you ask to check in with you in the days and weeks following the birth of your child? This can help you feel more like yourself versus the role of parenting that you just realized is overtaking everything else.

Have you communicated with your partner about how to best support you during this huge shift in life? What role or roles is your partner comfortable with during labor and after baby arrives? Some partners prefer to offer hand holding or emotional support and others like to help with tasks like bathing the baby or making dinner. Think about what your needs are and assign tasks to people. When I used to teach Sacred Pregnancy classes, one of the assignments I gave my students was to ask someone to make your dream meal for you after giving birth. That meal request can be handed off to the perfect someone who can make the dream come true. Truthfully, those nearest to you will be surprised and honored you asked.

DREAM TEAM STORIES

🗩 Liz Waid, former doula client and student

"I had my baby at home. After a few days of early labor contractions, it was finally time. From midnight to 2 a.m., my birth team showed up, consisting of my doula, my midwife, and my sisters. As they busied themselves setting up the birth pool, setting out supplies, my doula rubbed my back and followed me up and down the stairs to encourage labor while I hummed. It was a simple four note refrain over and over, low, and even. When everything around me was moving, the tune carried me on waves through the contractions, humming and breathing until the pain passed.

"When I could move to the tub, I felt relieved. We joked and talked for an hour or so as I sat in the pool. But, as the time got closer, I started doubting myself and my ability to let this baby enter the world. I asked to clear the room and just have my husband with me. I leaned over the side of the pool, tired and warm, as he sat outside it and faced me. He breathed with me and held my hands. He encouraged me. I was scared and I didn't want to push. I thought I couldn't do it anymore.

"When I went to push, I moved to the bed. I still didn't want to push, but my midwife was exactly who I needed her to be at that moment. She knew my abilities better than I did. I was still scared, but I knew my job was to focus. I felt a ring of fire and eventually I felt our baby release from my body in a great relieving rush. She was perfect."

📢 Affirmations from Amber Kilpatrick

"I am surrounded by a supportive and capable community. I will ask for help when I need it."

📋 Doula Wisdom from Kristin

Hire early. You will develop a stronger relationship with your dream team, and it will be easier to fit into your budget if you set up payment plans. We take clients last minute at Gold Coast, but it can be a strain on the pocketbook, and clients don't have as many choices if they wait.

CHAPTER 3

Deep Dive into Labor and Delivery Preparation

It is time to think about how you want to prepare for your labor and delivery, if at all. Some of my clients prefer to "wing it", as it suits their personality better. Others choose to take as many classes as possible, as well as read books and/or listen to podcasts. They want to soak in all the information. But do what is best for your budget, schedule, and personality.

Prepping your body for birth

I mentioned acupuncture, physical therapy, and Webster Certified Chiropractors as options to prep your body for labor. You can also consider using Spinning Babies techniques, or the Body Method Program. This information is found in our Resources section.

Fitness and Body Balancing

We asked Heidi McDowell to contribute this section on physical fitness during pregnancy, as well as the section on body balancing. Heidi is the owner of Mind Body Baby, a specialty yoga and barre studio in Grand Rapids, Michigan. She also is a former birth and postpartum doula with Gold Coast Doulas. Heidi is a Yoga Alliance E-RYT, a Registered Prenatal Yoga Teacher, Certified Barre Instructor,

Labor Doula, a Body Ready Method Pro, and has taken trainings with yoga teacher Jason Crandall and Gail Tully of Spinning Babies.

Physical Fitness

A growing body of research suggests that exercising while pregnant is beneficial, not only for a more comfortable pregnancy but also to help prepare your mind, body, and baby for labor and delivery. New parents often spend countless hours choosing the right items to add to their baby registry but can gloss over how important it is to find a physical preparation class led by a trained prenatal fitness expert. When taught by a professional, intentional movement can decrease or even eliminate common prenatal discomforts such as back pain, round ligament pain, fatigue, and incontinence.

During pregnancy, our bodies transform to accommodate our growing babies. As this happens, our posture shifts, we turn off essential muscle groups and often our core and pelvic floors are overly strained. Prenatal activity must be modified to accommodate, and more importantly, protect the changing body. Most providers would recommend shifting your exercise routine to a lower-impact option to reduce the risk of diastasis recti (abdominal separation) and pelvic floor bulging that could lead to an increased risk of tearing, or a pelvic organ prolapse.

Researchers studying the benefits of prenatal exercise found that at least 150 (minutes intentional, moderate activity per week resulted in a labor with fewer interventions, including a 35 percent decrease in the need for pain relief, 50 percent decrease in labor induction, 75 percent decrease in the need for operative intervention, and a 55 percent decrease in the need for an episiotomy.

Not all fitness professionals are created equal. A prenatal fitness expert has taken specific courses to educate themselves in the anatomy and physiology of the pregnant body to ensure the pregnant person and baby stay safe and free of injury. If they're passionate, they'll go a step further. See what related prenatal fitness trainings your instructor has taken before choosing your studio or class.

Yoga

Prenatal yoga is the most prescribed exercise by providers because of the intentional focus on physical and mental preparation. When taught by a Registered Prenatal Yoga Teacher (RPTY), a class becomes more than just modified poses to accommodate your belly. Each should include specific poses that strengthen, lengthen, relax, and balance the tissues of the pregnant body. It allows opportunities to quiet your mind and connect with your baby. Yoga teaches tools that offer comfort measures to use during birth, such as breath work, or pranayama, as well as self-trust, meditation, and surrender.

Childbirth education often is intertwined throughout classes filled with movements that transition into the birthing room. Yoga can fill your toolbox with physical and mental skills and offer a safe space to practice strong sensations. Prenatal yoga practitioners believe that you and your baby are the birth team, and by cultivating connection and awareness between the mind, body, and baby, you will develop trust in yourself and your instincts.

Yoga Contraindications

Some poses that should be eliminated during pregnancy are prone (belly down), supine (flat back) after 14 weeks, deep belly twists, intense core work, and breath retention. A RPYT should offer safe modifications.

Barre

Prenatal barre is a great option when pregnant because it has low to no-impact on your joints. Barre is a workout technique inspired by elements of ballet, yoga, and Pilates. Each barre class is designed to be a full-body exercise class that builds strength and endurance needed during birth. A class taught by a prenatal movement instructor would be highly modified and use bodyweight movements along with props for added resistance. During pregnancy, the center of balance is drawn forward with the growing belly. In these classes, poses are taught at the wall with the bar for support with a specific focus on the muscles needed to stabilize the pelvis and strengthen the core. A prenatal class will teach students how to engage their core to control intra-abdominal pressure and prevent bulging through the linea alba, which could lead to diastasis recti.

Barre Contraindications

Avoid intense core work, planking, jostling/jumping, heavy lifting, and deep twisting.

Swimming

Swimming is a safe, no-impact form of exercise for all trimesters of pregnancy. Being more buoyant in water is a great way to reduce the effects of gravity, taking pressure and stress off the body as your posture continues to shift with baby weight. Since balance can be impacted during pregnancy, surrounding yourself in water also minimizes your risk of falling. It's a good idea to move slowly when you enter or exit the water to avoid slipping. In fact, you might want to wear water shoes. Once in, swimming is a great way to maintain endurance and strength needed for childbearing and birth. Since there isn't limited impact on your joints, swimming typically won't exacerbate loosening joints. If you find your stamina beginning to wane in the third trimester, you can easily prop up on a kickboard for added support.

Swimming Contraindications

Avoid holding your breath while swimming underwater, twisting, and high temperatures such as hot tubs.

Regardless of how long you have been active, or of your level of physical fitness, all prenatal exercise needs a certain degree of modification to prevent injury to yourself or your baby. Each trimester brings a unique set of considerations. I would recommend using the internet to search for prenatal fitness professionals in your city. Speak to your friends or providers for referrals and recommendations. Sourcing online or live virtual classes is a great choice if your city does not have certified prenatal fitness professionals.

Consult your provider before starting any exercise programs.

Body Balancing
Contribution by Heidi McDowell

For me, body balancing during pregnancy is about being proactive versus reactive. Working with people during pregnancy is not only helpful for a more efficient birth with fewer interventions, but also is a path toward a more comfortable pregnancy. As a prenatal yoga instructor, my goal is to connect your mind, body, and baby. I want to help build strength and trust while cultivating a bit of inner peace. As a Body Ready Method Pro my goal is to identify imbalance in body tissue that could cause or lead to discomfort, delays, or interventions. I have combined my education to ensure people have prepared physically, mentally, and emotionally to help them meet their goals.

Our body's tissues hold the stories of our lives. Every trauma, every habit, and every pattern is mapped out in our soft tissue. The idea is to evaluate your body by looking at the posture, the gait, the body patterns, and determine which muscles need to lengthen, which need to strengthen, and, likely due to overuse, which need to just flat out relax. We want to create more space, more movement, and more function. We all know pregnancy is pulling and shifting the body out of balance. Often, we see the pelvis tilted forward, the glutes turn off, the pelvic floor being excessively loaded. Our bones, including the pelvis, are held by these tissues. Your baby will navigate the space provided, and if the optimal position for birth is difficult to achieve, it could be because your ribs are restricted or because your pelvis is tilted forward. In these situations, and others, a birthing person could experience delays starting or progressing through labor. The pelvis is not a fixed entity. It has four joints and can move, but only with the help of the tissue and extremities. We can change the shape of the pelvis to give baby more space during birth. The medical model of birth says when there's a delay, we need more force (think Pitocin). The physiological model says we need more space for your baby to navigate your pelvis and then maybe more force. What

42

is available to you during your pregnancy in terms of movement and positions is what will be available during birth. You don't jump off the couch and run the marathon, you prepare! Physical preparation during your pregnancy is as important as your childbirth education class and packing your hospital bag.

— Heidi McDowell

Childbirth Education

I took Lamaze classes with both of my pregnancies. I met other couples and enjoyed the time to connect with my husband after a busy workday. There are so many classes to choose from, too. You can take in-person comprehensive childbirth classes such as *Lamaze, Evidence-Based Birth*®, *Gentle Birth, HypnoBirthing: The Mongan Method*, or *The Bradley Method*. Some of these courses offer private options as well, in the form of virtual individual or group sessions. If you want a self-study class, consider our *Becoming A Mother* birth and baby prep course. You also should consider *Mama Natural, Birth Boot Camp, Birth & Baby University, Built to Birth*, or *Hypnobabies*. Some home birth midwives offer a custom home birth prep class that is specific to the needs of home birthers.

Many hospitals offer childbirth class options held on weekends and multiple evenings. Those classes can be covered by insurance but may not get into as much detail as the more comprehensive, paid childbirth classes. Some out-of-hospital classes are covered by insurance, and most are eligible for payment through non-taxed health savings and flexible spending accounts. Most classes include the partner or support person in the price of the class.

Other pregnancy and parenting classes to consider when preparing for birth and baby include multiples prep, siblings class, grandparents, cesarean prep, breastfeeding, back-to-work pumping, car seat safety, infant CPR/first aid, father classes, and classes to prepare a pet for a new baby.

Your area hospitals may offer some of these options. I would also do a google search to see if any area doulas, midwives, or childbirth educators have classes to offer in your area.

Even if you don't take a childbirth ed class, remember the principles of BRAIN

If you have hired a doula, they likely will discuss BRAIN.

BRAIN is an acronym for informed decision making in the event potential interventions are presented during labor. BRAIN stands for benefits, risks, alternatives, intuition, and nothing.

- **Benefits:** What are the likely benefits to making a decision to change course?

- **Risks:** Is my safety or the safety of the baby or babies at stake?

- **Alternatives:** Are there any options, and if so, what might we consider?

- **Intuition:** What does my "gut" say to do?

- **Nothing:** What if, as long as I am fine and baby is fine, we wait an hour?

Not Into Taking a Class?

No worries, here are my tips for other ways to prep for birth and baby.

Read books

Some of my favorite books include *HypnoBirthing: The Mongan Method* by Marie F. Mongan, M.ED., M.Hy, *The Birth Partner* by Penny Simkin, *Natural Hospital Birth: The Best of Both Worlds"* by Cynthia Gabriel, or *The Mama Natural Week-by-Week Guide to Pregnancy and Childbirth* by Genevieve Howland. We have a long list of book suggestions among the resources at the end of the book.

Look into Apps

My two favorite pregnancy apps are Wolomi and Expectful. Wolomi was created by a registered nurse of color for women of color to improve maternal outcomes with free and paid memberships. Expectful is a wellness and meditation app with support for fertility, pregnancy, and motherhood.

I also suggest installing Count the Kicks and a contraction timer app. Count the Kicks is an evidence-based stillbirth prevention campaign that provides information to parents and their healthcare team. I honestly don't have a favorite timer app, but I encourage you to check some out and pick one that works best for you.

Check Out Documentaries

Informed Pregnancy+ is a subscription streaming service with a focus on fertility, pregnancy, childbirth, and early parenting. You can find films like: *Business of Being Born, Trial of Labor, Orgasmic Birth: The Best-Kept Secret, Breastmilk*, and more. You can rent or watch any of these movies individually on various platforms.

Listen to Podcasts

Of course, our own *Ask the Doulas* podcast is our top pick as it has a mixture of birth stories and expert interviews. For birth stories check out the *Informed Pregnancy Podcast* and *The Birth Hour: A Birth Story* podcast. I have recently been listening to *The Happy Hour* with Bundle Birth Nurses as well. You can't go wrong with *the Evidence Based Birth®* podcast. I also love *Yoga Birth Babies*.

Create Boards on Pinterest

Are you a visual person? Then Pinterest is a great planning tool to consider. You can create boards for nursery planning, newborn sleep tips, baby registry options, birth planning, and more. Many doulas and childbirth educators share tips on Pinterest. You can look at the Gold Coast Doulas page for inspiration as well.

Look at Videos on YouTube or Vimeo

Platforms like YouTube and Vimeo have so much free content. You can find laid back breastfeeding demonstrations, paced bottle feeding, hip squeeze demonstrations, and even birth videos. Gold Coast Doulas has a channel with some great swaddling techniques and other helpful tips for clients.

Hospital or Birth Center Tour

A hospital tour or birth center tour is a great way to see the delivery rooms and ask questions. Some hospitals offer in-person tours and others only offer a virtual option. Even if you can't get an in-person tour, I recommend doing a test drive to the hospital and time out your route. Figure out where to park and ask if there is a different entrance in the middle of the night versus daytime hours.

Home Birth Prep

Looking into home birth preparation is useful for early laboring at home. Even if you are birthing at a hospital or birth center, you likely will labor at home for some period of time.

You may feel the need to clean or organize. This nesting instinct is an organic way to begin preparing for your new baby. If you slow down, you may enjoy this in-between time even more. Give yourself time to make sure you feel emotionally ready, and don't distract yourself with all the things you need to do or buy.

If you are having a home birth, your midwife will give you a list of items to purchase for your birth kit.

Birth kit Items to Consider

- Waterproof mattress protector
- Peri bottle
- Mesh underwear
- Thermometer
- Underpads or bed liners
- Bulb syringes

- Maternity pads
- Gauze pads
- Sterile gloves
- Receiving blankets
- Alcohol prep pads

I am a member of some home birth groups on Facebook where women pass along things to other home birthers that went unused from their kits.

If you want to birth or labor in water, some midwives rent birth pools or can tell you how to purchase one. I have had some clients purchase kiddie pools. There is one with fish on it that is quite popular for home births. Don't forget the hose you will need to fill the pool.

Some birth centers and hospitals also offer water births as an option.

Think about your space and prepping your bedroom and other places you want to labor to make them as calming, and distraction-free as possible. Use nesting time to declutter any areas you want to spend time. I am a big fan of using a yoga ball during labor. If you don't have one already, consider purchasing one. Your midwife may also ask you for a portable light source if you have dim lighting in your bedroom or other areas where you envision yourself being most comfortable.

Consider snacks for yourself and your birth team. This will keep you all going during labor. If it is a long birth, your midwife may appreciate having coffee or tea on hand. Think about things that you may want to eat after you deliver as well, particularly items that are easy to grab with one hand. One of my clients chopped up watermelon for after delivery and found it very hydrating and satisfying.

You also should consider packing a hospital bag in case of a transfer. And make sure your child car seat is installed properly and double checked.

If you already have kids, do you want someone to pick them up and take them somewhere? Sometimes doulas at home births are there just to offer sibling care. Will your pets need to go somewhere? Are they fine with visitors?

If you are birthing in the hospital, we discuss how to set up your environment in the next chapter focused on creating comfort.

What to Pack — The Birth Bag

Doulas often get asked by our clients what they should pack in their hospital bag. You honestly don't need that much, as most hospitals provide many of the items you will need, including most of what was listed in the Home Birth Prep section. Other items the hospital will provide include grippy socks, toiletries, numbing spray, pacifiers, diapers, a receiving blanket, nipple cream, a syringe bulb, petroleum jelly, and usually a fun or cute hat for baby. One thing to note is that if you want natural products for you or baby, it's best to bring your own.

Top Picks for What to Pack

For You...

Pack a gown if you don't want to use the hospital gown. They can be a bit awkward, and, well... breezy. You can purchase a labor gown online or look into the brand Pretty Pushers. Don't forget your insurance card. Bring the right office or work contact information. Include two copies of your birth plan, one for you, and one for your nurse. An eye mask could be helpful to get some sleep, a camera or phone to take photos or video, a charger for your devices, lip balm, snacks for after you deliver, hydrating drinks like coconut water or electrolyte drinks, essential oils if you use them, sticks of honey for energy, slippers with a grip, nursing bras or nursing tanks, a wireless speaker (if you want music, weather, news, or a podcast), going-home clothes, and your childbirth class manual, if you have one.

Other items to consider bringing are a nursing pillow, pajamas, or even a pillow and throw blanket from home.

For your partner...

The partner, family member, or friend who accompanies you during your birth likely will need snacks, a water bottle, toiletries, a couple of changes of clothes, a swimsuit if they plan to be in the shower, bath, or tub during labor. Extra socks is always a good idea. One of my clients brought a sleeping bag for her husband and he loved it. Slippers with a grip are also nice.

The partner also should have a list of friends and family members to contact with news of the birth. Some clients set up a group text or create a Facebook group to share photos, video, and announcements with friends and family.

For baby or babies…

Every newborn needs going home clothes, a swaddle blanket, an installed and checked car seat. Often the hospital or birth center will offer to provide ink footprints of the new baby or babies. The prints can be pressed onto a special piece of paper, and many people bring a baby book with space for footprints. Some clients bring special items for photos with their baby, like their name spelled in blocks, or something in the category of "hospital photo props" from Etsy. A headband or hat in baby photos is also something I often see.

Other Supplies

Many hospitals provide birthing balls, squat bars, and heat and cold packs. Some places now offer birth stools like the Kaya or inflatable birthing stools, like the CUB. A relatively new addition to labor and delivery is a type of inflatable pillow that the birthing person puts between their legs or leans into. It's formed in the shape of a peanut and is called a peanut ball. Just ask your nurse about these and other options.

The hospital will provide a hospital-grade breast pump, if needed. It may need to be used if a baby goes to the NICU. It's there if you choose to pump, or if you plan to exclusively pump.

Early labor signs

Here are some signs that are your body is getting ready for labor:

- Losing your mucus plug
- Having flu-like symptoms
- Surges that are similar to menstrual cramping or a tightening feeling your water may break in a large gush or a smaller trickle
- Upset stomach or diarrhea
- Feeling "off"

You will know if it is true labor when contractions get longer, stronger, and closer together.

What to do in early labor?

I tell my clients to think of birth like a marathon. You want to prepare for it by hydrating, resting, nourishing your body, and, if you want to think like a runner, do some visualization of your birth like you would for a race.

It is easy to get excited and try to get things going. Don't sprint, this is the time to conserve your energy. Take a nap, go about your everyday life until you cannot ignore the surges anymore and need more focus. Sit on a birthing ball and circle your hips. I love to tell my clients to go out into nature if the weather allows. Do whatever relaxes you.

The shower can be a great relaxation tool in early labor. The heat relaxes the muscles, and the water pressure can reduce discomfort in your back. Save the tub for when you are in more active labor, as it may slow things down in early labor. We will talk about comfort measures for labor in the next chapter.

When do you go to the hospital?

Here is the standard on hospital departure for a first-time mother. When surges are three to five minutes apart, lasting one minute in duration, and are happening consistently for one hour, it is time to go. Of course, that's assuming you're ready to go and within reasonable driving distance of the hospital. Always check with your medical provider on when they would like to see you, and factor in any additional logistical implications on your end, like sharing a vehicle, dropping off a child.

If you have two or more babies, you may want to adjust that to five to seven minutes apart, keeping your birthing history in mind, as well as the time it takes to drive to the hospital. The key is that surges consistently get longer, stronger, and closer together. Always discuss this with your provider in advance as far as their preference and when they want you to call their office and/or head to the hospital.

Final Birth Prep Wisdom from Kristin

Don't forget to set up childcare or pet care if you have other kids and/ or pets. You will want someone to be able to hear a call in the middle of the night if needed.

BIRTH PREP STORIES

💬 Elise Slade, former two-time doula client and student

"During my first pregnancy, my husband and I signed up for a Lamaze class. I was drawn to the formulaic nature of the methods we would be learning, thinking that it would be easier to use clear-cut strategies during birth as opposed to having to follow an instinct I wasn't sure that I even had. I learned a lot of valuable information in that class about the entire physiological process of birth and our instructor made all of the information easily digestible. There were two things that I found essential and valuable for labor preparation. The first was that every class we practiced tensing and relaxing different parts of our bodies as a way to prepare to relax through a contraction. The second was spending a lot of time in each class practicing different positions for labor. I found it very helpful to learn about what positions were going to help baby come down or help with the discomfort of contractions.

"Our time in Lamaze was very enjoyable. When it came to actually putting the breathing into practice during my labor, I found that I constantly needed my husband to cue me to do it. While this really made it a team effort, I found myself wishing that it had been more intuitive, the opposite of what I thought I would want! So, when I was pregnant a second time, I signed up for a hypnobirthing class. I absolutely loved hypnobirthing. I learned a completely new side to the physiological part of birth and enjoyed being able to expand my knowledge and perspective of the process from what I had learned in Lamaze. The best thing for me was listening to the affirmation track while I practiced self-hypnosis. It honestly gave me so much confidence going into my second birth. Everything about hypnobirthing was teaching me how to actually listen to my intuition and really working with my subconscious so that when labor actually came, relaxing was something that I could just do with a few very subtle cues.

"During my labor and birth I was able to fully relax between contractions, especially the pushing phase, and that allowed me to get good rest. I fully believe that it was what kept me from tearing, because I was able to relax my body so well. Both child-birth education classes provided me with invaluable information and strategies for coping with labor and I would wholeheartedly recommend either, it just depends on what kind of strategies you think you will be able to put into practice more easily."

📣 Affirmations from Amber Kilpatrick

"I love my wise, strong body."

📋 Doula Wisdom from Kristin

As your coach, I am here to tell you that you are strong. You've got this! When I went into labor each time, I loved to think about all of the women around the world who were in labor the same time that I was. I felt so connected and powerful. Make informed choices that are best for you and your baby or babies. If decisions need to be made, unless it is an emergency, you often have time to pause and ask questions. My clients tend to only have regrets if they feel that birth happened to them versus having an active role in decision making.

CHAPTER 4

Comfort Measures for Labor

Note: This chapter is not going to cover the stages of labor, nor will it have anything on interventions. We suggest you take a comprehensive childbirth class as mentioned in Chapter 3. In the following chapter, we are solely focused on your comfort.

Partner Communication

Your partner is key in keeping you comfortable in labor. They know you better than your doula, your mother-in-law, or other non-medical support team members do. It is important to find out if your partner has any fears related to the birth or caring for the newborn in advance of delivery. I teach a class called *Comfort Measures for Labor*, and in that class, partners talk about their feelings about birth and any fears they have. The birthing person also addresses any concerns. I discuss roles that the partner can play no matter the type of birth. This can include physical support, emotional support, helping with any decision making and for some women, just having their partner physically present is enough. It is important that the partner is flexible. I like to tell partners not to get offended as some of the comfort measures or coaching tools may work one minute and not the next. As doulas, we are never offended if our touch doesn't work or something we say is not motivating. We attune and take each moment as it comes.

Also, I realize that not everyone has a partner, and that many times a partner won't be at the birth. You don't need to have a partner to be supported.

Birth Preferences, Birth Plan

I am a big fan of a simple birth plan or birth preference sheet. It is an excellent discussion point with your provider as it gets closer to your due date. You can make sure that you are both on the same page. Many hospitals have their own templates that are easy to use, and childbirth classes often go through birth plans as well. It is helpful for nurses and other team members to know how to best support you. Be flexible and polite. Nobody likes a rigid plan as birth can be unpredictable. I suggest printing two copies for your birth bag and giving one to your provider at a prenatal appointment.

Here are two great questions to ask your provider during the birth plan conversation:

"Would there ever be a situation where you would override my wishes or act without my consent?"

"If you weren't on call when I go into labor would other providers in your practice be on board with my birth preferences?"

Things you may want to include in the plan:
- Name of your doula or team if you have one
- Goals and things that are important to you
- Things you want to avoid if possible
- Any newborn procedures you plan to decline
- Childbirth prep methods, if any, that your medical team should be aware of
- Environment (quiet, low lights, etc.)
- How you plan to feed your baby
- Anything else you want to communicate to your team

Your Birthing Environment

If you choose to give birth at a hospital, but still want the comforts of home, there are things you can do to make the experience less sterile and more calming. Birth is as mental as it is physical, so let's involve all the senses in preparing your space for the arrival of your baby.

Here are my top tips for making your hospital room cozy for birth:

Lighting

In nature, animals will seek out a dark and quiet place that makes them feel safe. This is because they are not threatened or disturbed. It is important for birthing persons to also feel safe to allow labor[19] to progress normally. Most hospital rooms have lights that dim, and you can request to have them turned down. Bring LED candles to add a lovely glow throughout the room, perhaps on the windowsill or in a bathroom. You could even consider twinkle lights for a pleasing effect.

Aroma

Some scents like lavender are known to have calming effects. Pack your favorite lotion or essential oil. Some hospitals do not allow diffusers, but you can bring one in case they do. Keep in mind that your sense of smell often is heightened during labor. I have my clients sniff a bottle of essential oil or favorite scent versus applying it directly. It can be disruptive if you can't get rid of the scent after realizing it bothers you. Along those lines, ask visitors to eat their food in the cafeteria or waiting room because even the aroma of bland foods can be overwhelming during labor. Remember, someone in labor changes their mind, and can change moods easily and often during labor. It's best to avoid anything that could be distracting in a time that requires quiet, calm, and focus.

Touch

Consider the textures of what you'll wear. You usually do not have to wear the hospital-given labor gown! If you prefer your own cozy robe or a long skirt and nursing tank, go for it. It can help you feel less like a patient and more in control. I feel the same way about bringing a pillow from home. It has your scent, the reminders of home, and will be much more comfortable than the common hospital pillow.

I advise you not to wear a tight sports bra during labor, it makes skin-to-skin contact with your baby or babies difficult, and there have been times when I've seen tight-fitting garments get cut off because they can be very difficult to remove with the number of tubes and wires involved in hospital births. Nursing bras and tanks are the way to go if you decide to wear something. I have had clients who birth in nothing at all!

Also, pack some hair ties or headbands to keep your hair out of your face.

Sound

You can't fully control the noises inside the hospital room, but you can influence them. Bring your own playlist of favorite songs to transport you to a calm place or change the mood to match the stages of labor. I have heard everything from classical music to reggae to rap at births. Some of my clients like to dance through parts of labor and others want a calming experience with softer music.

Guided meditations can also help you stay focused and relaxed. I personally love the Insight Timer app as well as the Expectful app for meditations. You can't count on your room always being quiet. Hospitals are typically noisy places. Bring a set of ear plugs or noise canceling headphones if you want to be able to create your own quiet oasis.

Your own voice and sounds can also create either comfort or stress. Vocal toning can be a great labor tool. It is the practice of making a low vibratory sound as breath is slowly released. It can be either a humming or a vowel sound that is slowly exhaled. I like to use the moo of a cow and as a doula I moo with my client. Remember if you are high pitched, you are going to create more tension. Tension=Fear. We want to create a relaxed state.

Sight

We often decorate our homes and desks with pictures of loved ones and our favorite art. There's no denying that having the sights of home and our favorite people around can provide support and comfort. Think about bringing something to focus on, like a family heirloom or personal keepsake. You don't have to go overboard in decorating a hospital room. Keep it simple and impactful with a few special items.

Do affirmations motivate you? Write out your favorites and hang a few up in the room. You can even purchase affirmation decks online from sites like Mama Natural. A sleep mask also can help you "tune out" when you need some rest or as a way to center yourself.

Taste

Hydration is so important during labor, but sometimes plain water doesn't seem too appealing. Bring an electrolyte drink or coconut water if those tastes are comforting to you. Honey sticks can be great tasking during labor, and also provide an energy boost. Sometimes a flavored lip balm and mints next to your bed can help throughout labor.

Hospitals tend to offer food options like ice pops, juice, broth, or Jell-O during labor. You also can ask for a cup of crushed ice. Crunching on a few pieces of ice can be satisfying and provide some hydration.

I would suggest that you eat something nourishing before going to the hospital or birth center. Top suggestions are…

- Scrambled eggs
- Oatmeal
- Bone broth
- Peanut butter toast (with a light spread of peanut butter)
- Brown rice
- Sweet potato
- Fresh fruit

- Juice pops
- Frozen grapes
- Granola, or a yogurt parfait

If you have health concerns, or particular dietary concerns, please talk to your provider and dietician.

Is Labor Really Painful?

What have you heard about labor pain? Are you getting your ideas from movies and television shows where the woman is screaming and everything seems out of control? Have you only heard fear-based stories from friends, or have you heard positive birth stories?

I had two unmedicated births. One was an induction with Cervadil due to preeclampsia, and one was a quick labor without any interventions that began on its own. I have a low pain tolerance in everyday life. Labor was not painful to me either time (other than the discomfort of back labor until my daughter turned) because your body gives you breaks to rest. It isn't the continuous pain of a throbbing tooth or an injured arm. I even see doula clients fall asleep during contractions and wake and get back into the flow of labor.

Let's get into some tools you can use for pain relief

Heat

Heat can be a great tool for relieving discomfort. You can use a rice sock, warm compress, a heating pad on medium, or a hot pack. Many hospitals have disposable hot packs that you can twist. I mainly use heat on the lower back to remove discomfort. It also can be used on the neck or shoulders.

You should not use heat on areas that are numb, or you could accidentally burn yourself. Sometimes you can get chilled during labor and a warmed blanket can be a nice treat.

A warm compress can prevent tearing during the pushing phase as well.

Cold

I love using a cold washcloth to relax my clients when they are feeling overheated during labor. I sometimes put the washcloth in a bucket of ice if she wants it to be really cold. The cloth can be used on the forehead, neck, upper chest, and even the feet during pushing. A cold washcloth also can help ease nausea. Some clients like the distraction of holding an ice cube in their hand as a way to reduce discomfort they are feeling from labor.

Physical Touch

Physical human touch can release oxytocin and reduce the perception of pain. Try slow dancing with your partner or utilize massage to help you through labor.

You can try light-touch massage, firm labor massage, counter pressure, hip squeezes, kneading, and more. Think about relaxing the areas of your body that carry tension like the jaw, forehead, neck, shoulders, arms, hands, lower back, legs, and feet. I use the double hip squeeze most frequently during labor as a comfort measure technique at the start of a contraction until it ends. It relieves the pressure on the sacrum and can give baby more room to move down into the pelvis. If you don't have a doula, you can find examples of what a double hip squeeze looks like through a simple web search.

Nerve Stimulation

Another option is to buy or rent a TENS unit. TENS stands for transcutaneous electrical nerve stimulation therapy. I don't have much experience with this and am not trained in this type of support, but many birthing persons have used this as a tool for natural pain relief. It is a small, hand-held machine that uses a mild electrical current to relieve pain. My husband has one for back pain and he says that it works well. Some doulas are trained to work with a TENS unit. Check with your provider before using.

Breathing

Breathing techniques are helpful to many women during labor. Yogic deep breathing is my favorite natural pain relief. It sends endorphins into the bloodstream and reduces tension, which then relieves discomfort. HypnoBirthing uses calm breathing techniques and birth breath during the pushing stage. Lamaze uses a technique called conscious breathing, which is focused on a deep, cleansing breath through the nose and an exhalation through the. We also learned a structured or paced breathing technique with shallow inhales and a long exhale. It was like a "hee, hee, hoooo". The biggest thing is that you want to focus your breath and avoid rapid breathing that may cause you to hyperventilate and need oxygen.

Your childbirth class may teach other types of breathing to use at different stages of labor.

Water

Hydrotherapy can be a fantastic physical and mental tool if you don't mind getting wet during labor.

The shower can be great during early and active labor to reduce discomfort and promote relaxation. The sound of the water running can help get you into a relaxed state as well as the heat applied to any areas that are carrying tension.

Many hospitals have bathtubs, and some have tubs with jets. You often can't deliver in the tub, but you can labor in the tub. If you are giving birth at a birth center or your home, you can likely consider delivering in a tub or birthing pool. Some hospitals offer water births as an option. As I mentioned earlier, save the tub for active labor so it won't slow down your contractions. I like to call the tub a natural epidural. It relaxes you and reduces the perception of pain. Many shower heads in the hospital are also detachable so you can use that on your lower back as well. It can also be nice to have your partner or doula take a cup of water and trickle it over your belly during contractions. It can be a relaxing ritual.

Some providers will offer sterile water injections for back pain relief. I have only seen this a handful of times, but it seemed to work well for my clients. The injections are said to cause a stinging sensation that wears off and can help you cope with labor pain.

Movement

Movement in labor is key. It can reduce the perception of pain. I tell my clients to listen to their body and move in the positions that feel good. We also talk about how you should change positions to keep labor progressing. It is a simple use of gravity and can speed up the labor process. (Simkin and Anchete, 2005)

Labor Positions

I discuss positions for labor in my Comfort Measures class. Here are some of my favorites.

Side-lying

Side-lying is a great position for rest, and you can alternate sides. This position can be used with or without an epidural. I suggest using a peanut ball or rolling up pillows to open the pelvis.

Sitting

A sitting position is great for rest, and it also allows gravity to assist. Seated on the birthing ball is one of my favorites as you can circle your hips and get hands-on support at the same time. It is a great position for giving double hip squeezes.

Use a chair or birthing stool. There are inflatable stools, called a CUB, at some hospitals. Sometimes there are wooden or plastic birthing stools available. Additionally, your hospital bed can be raised and lowered for some seated positions, like "the throne".

I am a big fan of toilet sitting. It can be uncomfortable, but it helps you make progress. The toilet is a natural place to relax and let go. You can sit facing forward or backwards leaning into a pillow on the tank.

Lunges

This can be done with a leg on a stool or as walking lunges. Lunges can aid with properly positioning the baby and open up the pelvis. Lunges are a tool doulas often use when labor stalls, provided the client has no medical or physical or restrictions.

Walking/Dancing

Some hospitals have rails in the hallways to allow for walking with stopping points to lean into the wall during a contraction. You can also walk around your birthing room. Dancing is one of my favorite upright positions. It is a great way for couples to connect and get oxytocin flowing.

Leaning

You can stand and raise the bed to lean into it. You can lean into the wall as mentioned earlier. You can lean into your partner.

Squatting

The squat is a great option if you are physically able with assistance. I like to take a sheet or rebozo and put it over a door or partner and support my client as they squat.

Kneeling

This position is great with support. I often see this during home water births with an inflatable birthing tub.

Hands and Knees

My favorite doula trick is to try hands and knees and have the birthing person circle their hips. You can set the birthing ball on your hospital bed and lean into it if you have someone supporting it. It is a great way to get some physical support like hip squeezes or counter pressure. I will never forget when my nurse demonstrated this technique during my first birth. I had back labor and I firmly believe that this technique flipped my daughter. My nurse walked out of the room and my daughter suddenly started crowning.

Note: Please consult your provider before trying some of the more physical positions like squatting or lunges.

Here are some labor or comfort measures reflections from women in pregnancy groups who were surveyed for the Beta launch of our *Becoming A Mother* course:

"Make sure the provider's goals are aligned with your own."

"I should have learned how to advocate for myself."

"I had no idea that labor would take so long and I would be tired."

"I wish I would have had a doula."

"I wish I would have moved more during labor."

"Wish I wouldn't have birthed on my back."

"I would have focused more on relaxation and massage."

"I had no idea that back labor was a thing."

"Birth can be empowering with the right tools."

"I wish I would have known about the risks and benefits of interventions, so I was more prepared to make decisions."

"I wish I would have known more about my options."

Positions for Birthing

Changing positions during the pushing phase can help align the baby properly and speed up the labor process. With help from a nurse, you can even change positions after having an epidural. Some positions can help reduce specific types of pressure or pain. Birth positions to consider include squatting, semi reclined, seated on birth stool (like the inflatable CUB), hands and knees, side-lying, leaning in a tub or against a wall, standing, or using a birth swing at a home birth or a birth center. Basically, you have options, and don't need to give birth in bed on your back. Just make sure your provider is on board. Check out *the Evidence on Birthing Positions* article from *Evidence-Based Birth* for more information. www.evidencebasedbirth.com/evidence-birthing-positions/.

Birth Outcomes

Birth is unpredictable. You can plan and prepare and still have a different birth outcome than you envisioned. One of the many things I took away from my doula training with ProDoula was that your birth outcome does not define your worth as a mother. Repeat that a couple of times to let it sink in.

This is not a competition. Well-meaning friends try to console you if your outcome was disappointing by saying something like at "least you have a healthy baby." Your feelings matter and are valid. You are allowed to feel disappointed if things don't go your way and you need to be heard to process and heal through it. I am a big fan of writing out your birth story as a way to process the birth and also have the memory for your child to experience one day.

BIRTH STORIES WITH DIFFERENT OUTCOMES

💬 Lexi Zuyddyk, former client and student

"When I became pregnant for the first time, I knew that due to my double uterus, a c-section was a very real possibility for me. I took Kristin's Sacred Pregnancy class, I chose an OB that supported my choice to attempt a natural delivery if possible, and with Kristin as my doula we created a birth plan that prepared me for both a vaginal or c-section delivery. Around 30 weeks, my OB informed me that I would be needing a scheduled c-section because my baby was stuck in breech position inside of my half-sized uterus and was now too big to turn. Despite being disappointed, I planned my gentle c-section to be as close to my wishes as possible and was even allowed to have Kristin in the operating room with me and my husband for delivery. Since I couldn't control the way in which my baby entered the world, I found peace in focusing on the things I could still control such as my determination to breastfeed and use cloth diapers. The mantra I chose during my pregnancy was 'Smooth safe birth, strong healthy baby' and in the end that was what we were blessed with!"

💬 Elise Slade, two-time doula client and student

"My first labor started with my water breaking in the middle of the night. I took a shower and contractions started, so I went on an early morning walk with my husband and tried to eat some breakfast. Active labor came within an hour. With my second labor, by the time I actually realized that it was the real thing, I was in active labor. My early labor contractions were all over the place and lasted for a few days (had some serious prodromal labor), so I was able to shrug them off as Braxton Hicks and go about as usual. I slept through my contractions becoming more regular until I couldn't anymore and realized that I was in active labor."

🗩 Sasha Wolff, two-time client

"As things started to intensify during my labor with my daughter, I started to lean heavily into my running background. As a runner who likes to compete against herself and others, I purposefully train to fight through the pain. Pain, to me, is both a mental and physical thing when it comes to running. There's a reason people say running is 90% mental and 10% physical. Our bodies are capable of SO much. We just have to remind ourselves of that. For me, when I'm running, I have to constantly reassure myself that my body can do what I've tasked it to. The same goes for labor. Billions of women throughout the ages have given birth. It's what our bodies are uniquely capable of. So, when I was in labor with my daughter and the pains started to sear through my abdomen, I told myself that 'Yes, it hurts now, but I will eventually cross the finish line called birth. At the end of this temporary pain, I'll get to meet my daughter.'

"Breathing also comes heavily into play both as a runner and a woman in labor. When running and things start to hurt, I start to calm down the panic in my head by breathing very purposefully. I employed that same technique during labor. With each breath in, I reminded myself of my strength and tenacity and with each breath out I repeated to myself that the pain isn't forever."

🗩 Katie Dykema, two-time doula client

"It was time to be induced and experience the magic I had heard about. We studied and practiced the Bradley Method Techniques. I had spoken positive affirmations to prepare my mind and body for what was to come. My sweet husband compiled my favorite songs into 'Katie's pushin' mix,' and my bag was loaded with LED candles, aromatherapy, homeopathic medicine, and other goodies to help aid and comfort during my labor process. Going into this life-changing event we knew we wanted a doula… and boy were we glad we made that vital decision. As first-time parents, we leaned on Kristin and her birth partner, Ashley, for advice, support, physical touch, encouragement and unbiased information. Will we do it again? ABSOLUTELY!

"After four-plus pokes to both arms while trying to insert the IV, I realized step-one of labor was to overcome my fear of needles. The Pitocin drip started… increasing one dose every half hour. Fast forward to 4 p.m. and I am at MAX Pitocin, and can barely feel the contractions. Truthfully, after a nap and all the talk of labor, I thought 'this is no big deal' (my water hadn't broken yet). After 10-plus hours, it was clear the Pitocin wasn't going to induce labor and our wonderful provider gave us the option to break my water or start reducing the Pitocin and begin again the following morning. We chose to break my water.

"With my water broken, the contractions started. They came on quickly and with intensity and seemingly endless peaks. Kristin gave me a tool— moo like a cow. Yup. The deepness in the vibrations helped aid our baby down the birthing canal. The more guttural I sounded, the more tension I could let go of. The experience was truly out of body, out of mind. My body felt it all, but my mind was able to separate and dig deep, knowing this was going to bring me the baby I had always dreamed of (gender unknown). My voice was quiet for most of labor and delivery. It gave me more concentration to do what I was told and let my body do what it was made to do. Our doulas gave us support and gave me the confidence and space I needed to conquer, strengthen, stretch, vomit, poop, laugh, cry, and slow dance endlessly, mooing into my husband's ear— over and over again.

"By 9 p.m., I'm considering an epidural. The waves were intense, overcoming my body and energy. It felt like we had a long way to go, but I knew the end was in sight. I can do this. I think…

"I hopped in the tub, which helped. We decided to lower the Pitocin and begin nitrous oxide afterwards. Whew. What a relief and beautiful way to aid in the comfort when I began to feel overwhelmed. The pain levels persisted but I no longer cared. We continued onward until it was finally time to push. Midnight came about the time Ashley arrived to take over in the crucial support role that Kristin had provided. Both Kristin, Ashley, and my husband used all their tools to support my physical body, while I simply imagined my hand raised to the sky, grasping onto God, and rolling with the waves. Although Kristin was supposed to be finished with her shift, she decided to stay by my side, and on the other side my husband was holding my hand and encouraging me. Meanwhile, Ashley was providing various much-needed modalities to keep me comfortable… running ice refills back and forth, massaging sore back muscles, and whatever other tools she had at her disposal. I had my own pit crew!

"Imagery, prayers, and faith kept me strong (while weak) and able to continue. For the next three hours it was on and I was quickly making the final push. But that pushing seemed to take forever and by 3 a.m. it was clear my baby's head was just not going to make it out. My OBGYN suggested an episiotomy. I truly was overjoyed with this option and said YES! A couple pushes later, they placed our beautiful baby GIRL on my chest! It was the craziest moment of my life. Utter shock, joy, exhaustion, hunger, and happiness. We did it! Our baby was healthy and it was time to 'rest' or so I thought. I didn't get as much sleep the first night, not as much as I had hoped."

📢 Meditation for Labor with Amber Kilpatrick

As your labor begins - trust your wise body.

Ride the intensity and the release of your contractions like a wave
Breath in - long and deep.
Breath out - with audible exhale.

Breathe.

Moan.

Roar.

In the space between contractions, notice your jaw—keep it soft. Notice Your hands—keep them soft. Notice your brow—keep it soft.

As your contraction builds, allow your body to tighten and squeeze as it harnesses all its power. Fill your body with a breath and open your mouth to let it out. This rush of air leaving your lips can be moans, groans, or screams.

Once your wise body has contracted, return to your soft jaw, soft hands, soft brow, and steady breath. Trust your wise body.

Prepare for the next wave.

📢 Affirmations for Birth with Amber Kilpatrick

I am a mother. A lion. A powerful force. I am ready.
I love my body and gain confidence in its ability to birth every day.
I deserve a positive birth experience. My baby feels my calm confidence.
I am in sync with my body and my intuition. My baby is the perfect size for me. I trust my body, my partner, and my birth team. My baby will be born easily and at the right time. I will breathe slowly and deeply to relax my muscles and bring oxygen to my baby. I am power-ful I am beauty-ful, I am knowledge-ful. I am in control of my pregnancy and the birth of my baby.

📋 Doula Wisdom from Kristin

Keep your movements smooth and in a rhythmic pattern and focus on your breath. Have your partner or support person remind you to change positions and provide feedback on areas of tension for focus, relaxation, and opening up rather than tensing.

CHAPTER 5

Lessons Learned from Birthing During the Pandemic

Gold Coast supported hundreds of families in the early stages of the pandemic. We found that one of the main concerns for new mothers was COVID, for good reason!

Women are resilient. We have always known this. Our clients have labored in masks, isolated themselves after giving birth, had visitor restrictions, and some were unable to have their doula with them in person.

We pivoted and so did our clients.

We found our clients still felt empowered with the judgment-free expert advice during birth and parenting, even when meetings and classes went from in-person to virtual. Their stories weren't always the same as some of the scary and heartbreaking tales that friends, the media, family, and even strangers told about their own births.

We were fortunate to work in a state where doulas were deemed essential, thanks to an executive order from Governor Whitmer's office. Many doulas in other states were unable to work for a year or longer. We worked through the entire pandemic other than for a few months in some smaller hospitals in our area that were only allowing virtual doula support. Our largest hospitals all considered certified doulas as essential workers. We showed our certifications to security, wore masks, and filled out a health evaluation form early in the pandemic.

Here are some important tips that we discovered first-hand while working with clients during the pandemic. Our feeling is that these learnings can just as easily apply during outbreaks of RSV, flu, and cold as well.

Tip # 1: Ask the Right Questions

Fear of the unknown is one of the biggest concerns we've heard from new mothers. Adding a wave of illness on top of those fears takes things to a new level. Here are the best questions we suggested our clients ask their health care provider while they were still pregnant!

What happens if I test positive for COVID?

What are the current visitor restrictions if any?

What happens if my partner has COVID when I go into labor?

If there aren't virtual tours at your hospital during COVID ask about parking and other instructions during this time.

Tip # 2: Set Boundaries

We know it can be hard to tell friends and family no. We don't want to seem rude or pushy, but it's important to talk to your partner ahead of time and come up with a plan. Will you allow visitors at home? What kinds of things will you consider helpful after your baby is born?

Ask for those!

Suggest virtual meetups and communicate ways friends and family can support you after baby arrives with meal plans, grocery store trips, gift cards for postpartum doula support, cleaning help, or a diaper service.

Tip # 3: Get Rest

Sleep is the best thing you can do for yourself each day. And it's free! Your body rejuvenates, cells repair themselves, and your immune system builds as you sleep. Try to get a full night's rest while pregnant. Work toward getting yourself on a good schedule before baby arrives. Once baby is here, track your sleep and make sure you're getting enough each day. Make sleep a priority, your mental wellness may depend on it.

Tip # 4: Keep Anxiety Low

Stress is bad for your immune system. Find ways to relax and talk to your health care provider about things that worry you.

What is relaxing to you?

Maybe it's reading, taking a warm bath, exercising, meditating, or going for a walk. When you feel yourself getting stressed or anxious, rely on methods to mitigate it that work for you. Find ways to laugh and enjoy time with your partner or friends.

CLIENT STORIES

💬 Birthing In a Pandemic, Samantha Veneklase, two-time Gold Coast client

"Due to the pandemic our birth plan was blown apart. It started with my husband not being able to go to appointments, having him drop me off at a completely different unfamiliar building due to offices condensing. I had to sit in a waiting room completely alone waiting to be called back to another room once again alone; it was so eerie. Leading up to our baby's birth we were dealt a lot of blows. Not only could we not have our doulas (at home or at the hospital, unless virtually), we couldn't have our midwife and it would be a team of strangers. Everything we planned for, even the 'unexpected', has been completely demolished and pulled out from under us.

"Getting to the hospital the day I was in hard labor. My mom dropped us at the door and was in tears as she had to just let us go in alone. We had to go through multiple screenings and checkpoints and ended up sitting in triage for two hours due to the hospital being short staffed. That was hard because I was in active labor and having a hard time. That was the hardest point for my husband because this was not how we expected it to go. We were supposed to have support and he really had the pressure put on him to keep me calm while staying in touch with our doulas to make sure they helped him help me. When we finally got up to our room, all the nurses and midwives were in masks, so I asked if I could see their faces because it helped comfort me more to put a face to the mask.

"I will say that aside from the chaos we endured getting up to our birthing room, once there and settled, we ended up feeling like we were in our own little bubble, and almost forgot about the pandemic going on in the world!

"The biggest challenge was after our baby was born... we planned to have a big announcement, our family waiting in the waiting room for my husband to go in and announce the gender, which in our case it would have been 'It's a boy!' We had plans for friends to come to the hospital as well to meet our baby for the first time, for a birthing photographer to be there through my labor and delivery and after to capture those precious moments we wouldn't be able to. Instead, we were alone, having to share the joy of our new baby with nurses and doctors and with family and friends through FaceTime. The happy joyful community moments we were counting on were robbed from us, though the one-on-one time with my husband and baby was wonderful, it was also at the same time lonely."

🗩 Meagen Coburn, two-time Gold Coast client

"Birthing in a pandemic. Not for the faint of heart, but like everything to do with motherhood, what other choice do we have but to go through it?

"April—Earth Day, to be exact—marked my second child's entrance into this chaos and my second childbirth experience with Gold Coast. With my firstborn, the fear of the unknown is the big cloud that hangs overhead. What is my body doing, what is my desired birth plan and experience, what is my recovery path? With a second child, you're empowered by experience. You've already earned your 'Mama Warrior' badge, you're in control. Your doula is really your friend, now, there to cheer you on during labor and delivery.

"But then a global pandemic changes all of that. Unknown viral transmission in public between people of all ages. Don't touch anything. Wash your hands. Children are affected, grandparents at heightened risk. And then, a statewide shutdown to 'Stay Home, Stay Safe'.

"There's no new-baby shopping. No pregnancy photo shoot. It's replaced with washing your groceries.

"My OB was placed at the hospital for the full last five weeks of my pregnancy, and ironically wasn't on shift when I delivered my son.

"Screenings into my office were mandatory. Did you contact anyone with COVID?

"Online check-ins became the norm to avoid registration counter services with the ladies I had grown to enjoy seeing every few weeks.

"Masks are mandatory upon entrance to all campus offices.

"Suggested inductions for mothers at 39 weeks, to limit time in-hospital in favor of laboring at home with a balloon induction.

"Removal of homemade masks in favor of surgical grade upon entrance to the hospital.

"Being held in triage for hours, while a room on the labor floor is cleaned to upgraded protocols.

"Meeting everyone in masks. I've never met the OB delivering my child, nor do I even know what she looks like.

"And the most memorable... pushing through delivery while still wearing that suffocating mask.

"Suddenly nothing about my pregnancy needs were for *me*. Everything I anticipated that 'I already knew' from my first went out the window. Many people don't know what a 'doula' is or means. For me, it's the difference between questions and confidence. Kristin, Ashley, and then ultimately, Julie, were my support network, my trusted news, my podcast resource, my answers, my cheerleaders. Everything I needed doula support for with this pregnancy was to understand *outside*, external and uncontrollable factors: can my husband come to the birth? What's the governor saying about my doula attending the childbirth?

"Are we doing this virtual, or together? What does childbirth look like in a hospital 'where all the germs are'? And through every question, every daily change in direction, and every phase of my pregnancy, labor, and delivery I was nothing but supported and brought a sense of calm despite the sheer chaos happening everywhere. Just like Julie physically holding my hand and telling me to breathe during the final pushes before my son was born, Kristin and Ashley were just as supportive to me emotionally through virtual resources leading up to this moment.

"While I may have completed my family unit with this pregnancy, I will forever sing the praises of doulas everywhere. Having doula support deemed an essential and allowable support service during a government lockdown truly proves exactly how essential it should be for mothers' consideration everywhere. Because Mama, you've got this, I promise. But you don't need to carry the weight of the actual world's problems on your shoulders alone."

📋 Doula Reflection from Kristin

Birth doesn't need to happen to you. Even if it doesn't turn out the way you dream, you can still be the hero in your own story. My clients are all heroes in my eyes.

CHAPTER 6

Newborn Procedures

Angela Tallon, M.D., is our expert contributor to the newborn procedures chapter. Dr. Tallon is a pediatrician practicing in Grand Rapids, Michigan. She owns Spirit Pediatrics. In addition to her experience in general pediatrics, she also has experience in the field of child abuse and neglect medicine. Dr. Tallon lives in Allendale with her husband and their six daughters. She has always wanted to be an author in any capacity and continues to pursue writing in her career.

If your baby is born in a hospital setting, there are a number of medical procedures that can be presented by hospital staff shortly after delivery. Some are offered to all babies while others are considered only in certain situations. Babies who have a need for resuscitation or urgent medical intervention at birth will be considered for these procedures when they are more stable.

Parents who seek information on these topics prior to their baby's birth will feel better prepared to make any decisions that are needed when the time comes. Parents who understand procedures hopefully feel more comfortable and confident making decisions, including in regard to some of the risks and benefits.

The Procedures

Circumcision

Circumcision is a medical procedure in which the skin covering the tip of the penis, the foreskin, is removed. In a hospital setting, it is usually completed upon parent request at some point before the baby is discharged from the hospital. Like any surgical procedure, circumcision has risks and benefits that are helpful to understand before making a decision to have a baby circumcised. Parents' reasons for wanting to circumcise their son can vary widely from primarily cosmetic/cultural reasons to religious reasons or medical reasons and beyond. Because this is a surgical procedure that permanently removes a portion of the human body, it's important for parents to consider their feelings about circumcision carefully and discuss their feelings about it prior to the birth. The most common side effect of circumcision is bleeding and, though rare, serious bleeding events occur.

Frenotomy

Frenotomy is another medical procedure commonly performed on newborns. It involves cutting the frenulum, which is the band of tissue connecting the underside of the tongue to the floor of the mouth. In some babies, this band of tissue is very short and tight, restricting the movement of the tongue to the point that feeding is affected, especially if the baby is breastfeeding. Cutting this band of tissue frees the tongue and often improves feeding. Again, the greatest risk of frenotomy is bleeding.

Hepatitis B

One of the three most common procedures performed on newborns is administration of the hepatitis B virus vaccine. This procedure often is performed very shortly after birth. The hepatitis B vaccine is the only vaccine routinely given in the newborn period and is typically is administered at the same time as the vitamin K injection is given and erythromycin ointment is placed in the eyes, which is discussed below. A person can have the virus but remain asymptomatic until liver cirrhosis or end-stage liver disease later in life. Because the hepatitis B virus can be passed from mother to infant during labor and delivery (though in utero transmission is rare), hepatitis B vaccination is recommended at birth to decrease the likelihood of newborns acquiring the disease.

Erythromycin Eye Ointment

The second of the most common procedures offered immediately after birth is the application of erythromycin ointment to both eyes. This is completed in order to reduce the risk of the newborn's eyes becoming infected with the bacteria that causes the sexually transmitted infection gonorrhea. This eye infection, if untreated, can be severe and sight threatening.

Vitamin K Injection

The third common procedure undertaken very shortly after birth is the vitamin K injection. Vitamin K, essential for blood clotting, is given to prevent vitamin K deficient bleeding (VKDB) that can result in increased bruising and bleeding. VKDB also can be fatal.

Researching Procedures Effectively

Because even well-known and well-respected online and printed medical resources differ widely in the way risks and benefits of the above procedures are presented, it isn't possible to identify one recommended resource that could serve all parents' educational needs. Instead, it is encouraged that parents use the process of researching infant procedures as a means of becoming familiar with different medical websites in order to discern which one(s) they prefer. After baby's birth, it will be important that parents have websites that they trust to look up basic information about infant care, medical topics they're interested in, or minor concerns they have between doctor visits. It is important that parents visit the "about" page on any website in order to better understand the quality of the information provided on the website and any biases that might be inherent in the content presented.

Examples of quality websites for learning more about the above newborn procedures:

- WebMD.com
- Mayo Clinic
- UpToDate (Patient Education section)
- HealthyChildren.org

Examples of quality websites that present some alternative viewpoints on these topics:

- DoctorsOpposingCircumcision.org
- Medela.com (frenulotomy)
- Alternative medicine and holistic health websites

Above all, it is important to realize that learning on the internet can be fraught with pitfalls. It also is the reason so many parents are able to become more knowledgeable on medical topics than ever before. It is important for parents to put all the fruits of their research into perspective in order to make the decision that is right for their baby and the family. As always, if you are overwhelmed by the process or have specific questions, it's a great idea to involve your baby's physician. Schedule a visit with him or her just to address your questions and concerns. Many practitioners are open to this approach and appreciate the time to get to know parents even before the first visit with the baby and/or touch base with parents already established in the practice.

NEWBORN STORY

💬 Marta Johnson-Ebels, former doula client

"I was both terrified and in shock when I learned that my daughter was born with congenital heart disease. If she was going to live, she needed surgery. Having lost my two previous pregnancies and not knowing how much medical treatments had advanced, I had no idea what to expect in terms of her survival. Thankfully, Helen DeVos Children's Hospital has surgeons who are top in their field and have excellent bedside manner. They included me in discussing her care, explained risks in a way that was straightforward and accessible for those new to serious surgeries, and even drew pictures to fully explain her condition and what was going to be done to fix it.

"Claire ended up spending 77 days in the hospital, most of those days in the ICU. We got a little break after her first surgery. I am thankful we were able to get a little routine and some days without tubes in her nose and mouth. I felt like I got to know her a little bit before her big heart surgery. Her PICU rollercoaster felt totally outside of my skill set. Taking part in her morning rounds, asking lots of questions and doing tons of reading on heart babies helped me regain my confidence. I kept a really close eye on her and one day I was able to notice that she didn't respond to suctioning like she normally did. I raised an alarm with the nurse, and they did testing and found that she had clots everywhere. She was diagnosed with a blood clotting disorder and was put on blood thinners. I felt like I did something in that moment that made a difference as a mom. From then on, I felt more confident in my 'mom instincts'."

📋 Doula Wisdom from Kristin

If something feels "off", follow your mom instincts and talk to your pediatrician or get a second opinion. Nobody knows your baby the way you do.

PART 2

Baby Prep and Setting Yourself Up for Postpartum Success

CHAPTER 7

Postpartum Planning

How will you survive? Setting yourself up for postpartum success.

Let's start by defining postpartum because I hear it used incorrectly all the time. Someone will tell me, "I had really bad postpartum" or "I really struggled with postpartum after my second child."

Postpartum does not equal depression. Postpartum literally means a period of time after childbirth So, you may or may not have struggled with postpartum depression, postpartum anxiety, postpartum weight gain, postpartum hair loss, or any number of things that can happen to a body after pregnancy and delivery. But everyone who has given birth has been through the postpartum time, the period of time right after having a baby. It sometimes is referred to as the fourth trimester and has nothing to do with depression.

I will discuss perinatal mood and anxiety disorders later. I just wanted to make it very clear that when I mention the term postpartum, I am not talking about mental health.

Communication

Some of us are really good at communicating and some of us maybe think we are... but what would our partners say? Communication is a skill. If you don't consider yourself to be a good communicator, luckily, it's a skill that can be learned. A therapist is actually a great place to start. Find out what's holding you back, what are your barriers, and how you can overcome them?

Why is communication so important? When this little human (or these humans) enter your life, it will be chaotic for a while. Setting clear expectations ahead of time will save you unnecessary and unwanted arguments with yourself and likely your partner later.

How do you set clear expectations? Be clear in your requests; don't make them vague. Our partners usually cannot read our minds.

Express what you need. Don't be afraid or ashamed to ask for help.

Be easy on yourself. Don't hold yourself to unrealistic expectations.

If you have a husband or partner who is involved in your life and your soon-to-be child's life, prioritizing that relationship is very important. Now, while you're still pregnant, talk about this together. How will you prioritize your marriage/partnership/relationship?

Talk about how your relationship might change in good and bad ways. Be prepared. Here are some examples of possible scenarios.

Some couples become closer after a baby is born. You may find that your partner really embraces this new parenting role, and it makes you love them all the more. They're super helpful, they listen, and they do whatever they can to help.

Your partner may feel left out after the baby is born, especially if you are exclusively breastfeeding. If you have a partner who wants to be really involved, it may feel like there's nothing for them to do in the beginning. Mom, it is up to you to change that. Talk now about all the things your partner can do to help.

Here are some the duties partners often take on.

- Changing diapers
- Settling the baby into the crib for naps and bedtime
- Bringing you snacks and water while feeding

- Hanging out with you while you feed
- Giving the baby a bath
- Snuggling with the baby to give you a break to nap or shower
- Spending dedicated time with an older sibling

There are so many ways a partner can be involved and connect with the baby.

Your partner may feel neglected because the baby gets all of your attention. For this person (you know who they are if you have a partner like this), I suggest talking over the same list we just mentioned. Make sure they understand that you are the one who needs attention right now, not them. Do this while being mindful of your partner's needs and finding a happy medium. We don't want anyone to feel neglected, but in the initial postpartum weeks it's all about Mom and baby.

You may feel resentful that your partner gets to leave, go to work, and go about their day as normal. You feel stuck at home doing the same thing over and over again, like the movie *Groundhog Day*. Some mothers will never feel this, and for others it's one of the hardest parts of parenting. It will be important to find ways to do things you need and want to do as well. Letting your partner know if/when you feel this way is important. Otherwise, they may think you're happy with your routine at home. Find ways to have some alone time, to get out of the house, meet a friend, whatever you need to do. But try not to feel angry and resentful that your partner "gets" to go back to life as normal. Again, a therapist can be really helpful here.

When I was an active postpartum doula, I remember a client of mine venting to me during a shift. While she sat on the sofa in her three-day old sweatpants, hair a mess, breastfeeding her baby, she was so angry that her husband got to leave every day. "He gets to wake up and shower, pour himself a cup of coffee, and drive away to work every morning. By himself! He can drink his coffee and listen to music or a podcast. Then he gets to go out to lunch…"

You get the picture! This mom felt trapped at home, and she was becoming very resentful. We slowly worked on getting her baby into a consistent feeding schedule so she had longer stretches to herself and the chance for more time to leave the house while her husband could stay home and care for the baby with a reduced concern about feeding intervals. I remember the first time she left the house to get a coffee, she texted me thrilled as she sat alone at the coffee shop! All while looking at photos of her baby, of course!

So, be open and honest with each other. Talk about your hard days and let your partner know how they can best help. Don't let an issue build until you're so frustrated that you blow up and yell. We've all been there, and it does no good.

Define Household Roles

Defining household roles while pregnant also can be helpful. How do you currently split chores? Who will get groceries and make meals? Who will do dishes, laundry, and clean? Do you have the means to hire help? If not, do you have a friend or family member who could help in those initial weeks?

Do you have older children? Who will care for them and get them to school, sports, etc? Are your children old enough to help with chores around the house? If so, make sure they have their own set of responsibilities. Depending on their age, this often makes them not only feel helpful, but to be very important in this time of change. It feels good for them to know they are doing something for the family that maybe only they can do.

Do you have pets? Who will make sure they are fed, walked, and taken to vet appointments?

Who will be in charge of making sure you don't run out of diapers and wipes? Create a station or stations around your home and keep them stocked. Stations are great in multilevel homes so stairs aren't walked up and down as often.

Who will be in charge of making sure bottles and/or pump accessories are clean and stocked? These will be used multiple times a day for a mother who is pumping and bottle feeding. Keeping up with cleaning bottles and parts can be a never-ending battle.

Will you need help in the yard? Who mows the lawn, shovels the driveway, and picks up dog poo in the yard? Do you have a garden that needs to be planted or tended?

Find the Help You Need

If you don't have a partner, setting up a support system ahead of time is even more crucial. Who do you have that you can rely on? Will they help out during the day or overnight? Can you hire a postpartum doula? If you're having a baby shower, consider asking for help instead of stuff. Oftentimes doulas provide gift cards for overnight care or lactation support. Ask for gift cards to your favorite restaurants so you can order food. Ask for two cleaning sessions a month from a professional company. Think of ways you may need the most help and incorporate solutions into your gifting options.

If you are on bedrest, or think you may end up on bedrest, see if you can find a local bedrest doula for support. Otherwise, find a trusted friend or family member to help. If you end up on bedrest, you may not be able to finish organizing, put away baby gifts, or set up the crib.

Set Expectations

So, we covered communicating with your partner, but what about communicating with everyone else? Communicating with our friends and family can be dreadful. Our experience dealing with the COVID pandemic made things even more tricky. We used to just worry about people visiting during flu season, but I think for most of us, living through a pandemic opened our eyes to a lot of things.

Pandemic or not, as new parents you will have to decide who you will allow in your home, and when. Are vaccines important to you, and if so, which ones?

Will visitors have to wear a mask? Will they have to remove shoes before entering, wash hands before touching the baby? Will you only allow visitors at certain hours of the day? If your friends or family members have children, are they allowed to visit, too?

These are all very personal decisions, and there is no right answer, only what is right for you.

Talk through different scenarios together so you know how each of you feels, and try to stay consistent. Be clear that the rules are for <u>all</u> visitors so nobody thinks they are being singled out.

Is there someone you do not want to visit you? Make sure you talk about this before your partner invites them over.

Unfortunately, after you have a baby, there will be people who won't listen to what you ask of them. They may even hear you but disregard what you say you need or want. They will tell you what they think you need or want. Tread carefully here so as to not offend, but make sure to stand your ground and that your partner has your back. They should be able to help shut down negative conversation, change the subject, tell the person their comments are unwelcome, or ask someone to leave, if necessary.

Visitors can be exhausting. Everyone wants to come hold the baby, which isn't usually very helpful. You end up playing host, making them coffee or tea, and talking while they hold your baby. You'd rather be taking a nap or a shower, eating a meal, taking a walk, or running to Target alone; anything but sitting there hosting a guest while they hold your baby.

Be clear. Let people know what you need. If someone wants to visit, let them know they may visit, but that you need lunch or you would love it if they could do dishes and fold laundry while they are there. Have a to-do list on the counter they can look at if you're comfortable doing that. Not many people will tell a new mother no if you ask for help when they visit.

It's OK for you to say no! Visitors can be stressful. You never know if your baby will be nursing or tired. Someone always arrives just as your baby goes down for a nap and then you feel obligated to get the baby up so the visitor can see them. Or someone arrives right at feeding time, and it takes you 45 minutes to nurse. Most moms, especially new moms, are uncomfortable nursing in front of friends and family, and even if you are, your visitor might be made uncomfortable.

A friend of mine told me the other day that as a new mom, all these family members would just show up at her house all the time. One day there were several people over, and the baby needed to be fed, so she told them she was going upstairs to nurse. Once in the nursery, she took her shirt completely off because the baby was fussy, and she was still struggling with breastfeeding. It was much easier to nurse topless than mess with covers and nursing shirts or bras. So, she's sitting in the chair topless, feeding her baby, when a couple family members walk in (the door is closed mind you!), sit down, and start chatting with her. She said she remembers feeling like she wanted to burst into tears. She felt so overwhelmed. She just wanted peace and quiet and to be alone with her baby while he fed, and her family members didn't respect her request.

Visitors can also be difficult because you don't know what your own energy level will be a week, a day, even a few hours ahead of time. You can't anticipate how you'll feel on Tuesday at 1 p.m. when Aunt Jan is coming to visit. If you are too exhausted for a visitor one day, it's OK to cancel. Or, let Aunt Jan come and tell her you're exhausted. She can come watch the baby and put away dishes while you nap.

For others, pregnancy is all about you and postpartum is all about the baby. Most people will not think of you first. Find your people, the people who do think about you and want to help and let the rest of them wait until you're ready to see them. Don't feel like you need to entertain. You're not obligated to do anything for anyone other than yourself and your baby.

Take as much time as you need to figure out this mothering gig. Cuddle with your baby. Take naps and stay in your pajamas all day. Lie in bed with your partner and talk about what an amazing human you created.

Fourth Trimester Preparation

Plan for postpartum as much as you do for birth! We spend so much time following apps that tell us what size our baby is, researching different diaper brands, or finding the perfect crib—all the very cute and fun aspects of pregnancy—but most parents bring their baby home that first day and realize they didn't spend any time on what to do now!

You obviously can't plan for everything. Some of this you will figure out as you go, but here are some of the major pain points and things to set up before your baby arrives.

Postpartum Supplies

There are some supplies you may want to consider for use after delivery. Some of them I've used, and some are ones that clients and students have mentioned over the years.

Pads or adult diapers

If your water breaks at home, you'll need them until you get to the hospital. Even if you have a home birth, it may be hours until you give birth, and you'll want something for leak protection while you wait. You'll also likely need them after delivery as you may have some discharge and blood for two to three weeks or so; kind of like a light menstrual period.

Hospital supplies

Prepare to have some mesh underwear and a peri bottle or two, perhaps from the hospital. Depending on where you deliver, you may get to take these home. Again, the mesh underwear and pads will collect any blood or discharge. The peri bottle can be filled with warm water and squeezed while you urinate to help with any burning. It also is helpful with cleanup.

Stool softener

Pooping after giving birth can be a scary thought. Ask your doctor about taking a stool softener and make sure you're eating enough fiber. In other words, eat your veggies! The last thing you want to do after giving birth, especially if you've had any tearing or stitches, is push too hard during a poo. Hemorrhoids are not a pleasant experience after giving birth either. Ask your doctor about recommendations for those, as well, if you've found that pushing has caused some angry spots in the butt region.

Nursing bras or tanks

These can be handy in the hospital, especially a tank. Wear the tank or bra once you can change out of your hospital gown. It makes for easier breastfeeding. You'll use these a ton at home, and to nurse in public, too.

Meals

The last thing you have the time and energy for when you have a newborn is cooking. We talked about this a bit before but look into local meal delivery services. If there's nothing local, there are several national delivery options. Many of them offer great deals for first-time subscribers. Also ask friends who use meal services for a coupon code.

Frozen meal prep

If you like to cook, think ahead, and fill your freezer with easy to heat meals. Make sure they are nutrient-dense with lots of protein and veggies. If you have a deep freezer, fill it!

Meal trains

If you have a group of friends or family that would put together a meal train for you, there are websites that make it really easy (just search meal train websites). If you have any food allergies or sensitivities, be sure to let them know and request specific meals if you prefer. You can also ask for meals from restaurants or gift cards if homemade meals freak you out.

Grocery delivery service

Look into what local grocery stores offer delivery or easy pick-up service.

Find easy recipes

Talk to your friends and ask them for the easiest recipes they have and start a collection. Cook crock pot meals ahead of time that can be easily reheated for a second meal.

And always remember, when someone asks if they can bring you something, accept food.

Childcare

It seems strange to think about childcare during pregnancy, but many childcare centers have a waiting list. You will need to take into account how long your maternity leave is, if you work out of the home or not. If so, will you return to work? Part time, full time, work from home, stay home? No matter what, you will need to budget for your choice.

Maternity Leave

How much time will you take off? Do you want to find a daycare center, an in-home daycare provider, or hire a nanny in your home? Maybe you have a parent or grandparent who will watch your baby. Are there childcare centers located conveniently between home and your place of employment? Consider location, convenience for drop off and pick up, and make sure to do a walk through first. Ask all of your most pressing questions to help understand whether or not you would feel comfortable leaving your baby there.

Does your partner have leave from work to help at home, at least initially? Who do you trust to help you in those critical first weeks postpartum? Who will actually support you and listen? You need help and support from someone you trust. Are there local postpartum doulas in your area? They often are available to work days as well as overnight shifts. Do you have family or friends who will be helpful? Set up a plan now so you know you have support once you get home with your baby.

Cleaning

Will you get help from a housekeeper? A family member? A postpartum doula? Will your partner clean? If the answer is no to all of those, feel free "nest" all you desire before the baby or babies arrive, but once you've delivered just leave the house as-is for a while. You need time to recover, and a tidy house is nothing to stress about in those early postpartum days.

If you're the type of person who gets stressed by a messy house, this will be an important point for you to figure out before your baby arrives!

Baby Showers and Baby Sprinkles

Register only for the necessities. You don't need all the hype. Most of the items you think you need, you will never use. If you find you need it, you can purchase it later. Many times, parents purchase things they never use, buy clothes that never fit, don't have time to return them, and end up wasting money.

I mentioned it earlier, but if you register for help (overnight support or meals, for instance), that will help you tremendously in those initial weeks. See if any local doulas offer gift certificates. You can ask your friends and family to put money toward birth or postpartum doula support rather than more outfits or fleece blankets.

Find local shops to support when possible. It's so easy to find items from the big box stores, and when you're a busy parent trying to build a registry, this is really convenient and easy. But if you have local stores that you can support, see if there is a way to add them to the registry, or put a gift card to their store on your registry. Even the smaller and independent stores have ways of doing this now.

Without getting too specific about products, I do want to make some suggestions on items to consider when creating a registry. When talking with soon-to-be parents in the classes I teach, there are always a lot of questions around what to buy and what not to buy. Obviously, we won't agree on everything, and what one family finds necessary another may find useless. My best advice is to keep it simple. Like I mentioned earlier, you can always buy or borrow what you need later if you don't have it.

Necessities

The Seat

A car seat is a must. Do your research and find a car seat that works for your car and your family.

What's important to you? The weight of the car seat? If it transfers to a stroller? Is it safe for preemies? Side a note here, car seat selection, not to mention the seat itself, can be extremely confusing. Most cities have certified car seat safety technicians[20] who will show you how to properly install a car seat. You'll want to adjust seat settings with each new stage baby development. A big change is when your baby or babies grow enough to begin riding in a front-facing seat rather than a rear-facing seat. In fact, consider getting a small mirror for the back seat headrest of your vehicle while the child is still in a rear-facing seat. The mirror facing your child allows the driving using the rear-view mirror to see the babies face. This way you can see if your baby is upset, has spit up, is gagging on something, or what have you. Otherwise, you will be in the car peering at the top of your baby's crown simply guessing on what's happening back there.

The Bum

Another primary considering is whether you use cloth or disposable diapers. And wowza, you will go through a lot of them. You'll get so good at changing diapers you'll feel like you could do it blindfolded. Actually, you will be able to do it blindfolded. There are tiny little newborn diapers with a cutout for the umbilical cord that you may want to consider for the first couple weeks, regardless of how you diaper. Often, the cloth diapers are really big on a newborn. If you don't have a membership to a bulk store you may want to get one to save money on this one item alone. They will typically have a store brand for disposable diapers along with name brands. Same with wipes. You'll need a lot of those and you can typically purchase them in bulk to have plenty on hand and save some money. There also are subscription diaper services that provide what is required by delivery on schedule with your baby's development. Some popular subscription services are The Honest Company and Coterie.

Those Baby Clothes

Purchase minimal clothing. You will probably change a newborn's clothing a few times per day. They poop, pee, and may puke often. If you do laundry once per week, you'll need enough clothing to get you through seven days. That's nearly 30 outfits, if not more. If you do laundry more often, you'll need fewer outfits. Keep in mind that babies grow fast. Don't over purchase because before you know it, they won't fit into all those cute, little newborn outfits. They hang in the closet never worn.

Bottles?

If you are not breastfeeding, then bottles will be necessary. They may be necessary even if you're nursing your baby or babies, if you're pumping to store mother's milk. Anyhow, there are so many different brands and types of bottles that it would be impossible for me to tell you which one is "best". You may have to try a few to know which one or ones your little one prefers.

The Crib Business

A crib or bassinet is necessary for optimal sleep and safe sleep. If you are breastfeeding, a bedside bassinet can be ideal, so you don't have to get out of bed to feed, and your baby has its own flat, safe space to sleep. Most parents aren't ready to use the nursery immediately. They feel strange having their newborn in a crib in another room. You may move the crib into your bedroom for a while if you have the space. Either way, you can sleep soundly knowing your baby is nearby and sleeping on a flat, safe surface.

Look at that. I only have a few items on my necessary list. All the rest is extra. Your baby probably doesn't need much else, so the more you add to the list the more complicated things can become. If you register for some necessities and then get the rest in gift cards (to use later on what you actually know you need), food, and postpartum support you're golden.

The Extras

Here I will share some optional items that I think may be worth your money. I'll cover some of these optional items in greater depth in the chapter on sleep, but a sound machine is a near-must for me. It is helpful, particularly in the first six months. That static sound while sleeping will really soothe your baby and help keep them asleep longer. You also can consider a portable machine if you travel a lot. It can be used in hotels, or even in the stroller.

I mentioned that babies pee and poop a lot. This is true. Many of these events happen overnight, sometimes leaving sheets and possibly the crib mattress soaked. I recommend buying two or three waterproof mattress covers. Why so many? Because if this happens more than once in a night, you need backups. The last thing you want to be doing at 3 a.m. is washing crib sheets and cleaning mattress covers to put your baby back to sleep. You just strip the crib of the wet stuff, wipe it down, remake it with clean covers and sheets, and maybe rinse the soiled stuff but otherwise bother with laundry in the morning.

Swaddling blankets and/or sleep sacks are wonderful. Again, there are a ton of different brands and types, but every baby seems to have their own preference. The point of swaddling is to hold the baby's arms down while sleeping and make them feel snug and safe, like they felt in the womb. Swaddling with a blanket usually works during the newborn phase, but once your baby wiggles more and gets stronger, they can usually push their way out of even the best blanket swaddle. Of all the clients I've worked with in this area, some of the favorite products have been the Miracle Blanket, the Love to Dream Swaddle, The Butterfly Swaddle, and Swaddelini, which a local woman-owned business and Gold Coast client.

Bibs are good for all the spit up. This way you're only washing bibs instead of entire outfits.

If you plan to baby wear, a sling or carrier is a must. Again, you'll need to do some research and decide on one that works best for you. You may find that one is too confusing, and another one is uncomfortable or too heavy. If you are able to test some out before spending the money, do it. It's also wise to hire a babywearing consultant if you have one locally. There are wrong ways to wear a baby, and, as your baby grows, most slings have to be worn another way to keep your baby safe.

More than likely, you will opt to purchase a stroller. I swear, besides the car seat, this is the toughest decision most parents make for their postpartum journey! Go to the store to feel the strollers and push them around. Does the handle adjust if you or your partner are tall? Does it fold easily? Is it too heavy? Is it too small or too bulky? Do you need one that will grow with you as your family grows? Do you want a jogger? If you're having multiples, you'll probably want a double stroller. This is a completely personal decision that only you can make based on use and budget.

If you plan to breastfeed, somewhere along your journey you will likely need a good breast pump if you ever want to leave and have some-one else feed your baby. If you have multiples, babies in the NICU, or decide to exclusively pump for any number of reasons, you will need a breast pump. Get a recommendation from your local International Board Certified Lactation Consultant, if there is one in your area, or ask in your breastfeeding class. Don't forget to check with your insurance provider to see if you get an electric one for free. There are also hand pumps that are easy to bring along for short trips.

Nursing pads can be helpful if you leak. Typically, most moms leak in the early stages of breastfeeding, and even if you don't breastfeed there will be leaking as you let your milk dry up. If you do leak and don't use nursing pads, you could get wet spots on your shirt, which can be a bit embarrassing and uncomfortable. There are milk collectors you can look into. I used them initially when I was breastfeeding, but I found them to be more of a nuisance than saving a bit of extra milk was worth!

I love bouncy seats. Once your baby is big enough to sit in one and kick their little legs around, they have so much fun! Purchase a basic one. You know, the rounded metal base with a cloth seat. There's no need for the fancy ones that make noise and move in 18 different directions.

Diaper pails don't become necessary for a little while if you exclusively breastfeed. A breastfed baby's poo doesn't usually smell, so a pail is really not necessary until they start eating solids or if you use formula. Then you'll need one to keep the stink contained! Diaper pails do have an insulating seal around the top to reduce smell from escaping. In the meantime, you can just use a regular old trash can and empty it every couple of days.

You will probably want baby nail clippers. Eventually their nails will get too long, and some babies are even born with long, sharp fingernails! You'll want to do this in a well-lit room and don't cut them too short.

If you breastfeed, Lanolin cream, Nipple Butter, or some sort of balm for dry or cracked nipples may be needed. You also could look into nursing cups or shields that protect your nipples. The damage could be a result of your baby's latch, so if you see your nipples cracking if you feel them becoming extremely painful, reach out to your IBCLC for more support.

A baby bathtub is really useful, and fun! Where you plan to bathe your baby—in a sink, bathtub, or shower—will determine what kind of tub you need. There are many designs for the many different uses.

You'll likely want a diaper bag for outings. There are a ton of cool ones, just pick one that is functional as well as stylish. Some even have insulated pockets or coolers for milk. Whether you like big bags or backpacks, you can find the right one for you. Sidenote here, it's easy to forget things when you head out for the day with your baby. You might consider making a checklist of everything you need in your diaper bag.

This task is something that could be given to an older child or your partner. Ask them to always keep the diaper bag stocked and ready so all you have to do is add milk or formula before you head out the door. Getting somewhere and realizing you have no diapers, wipes, or a change of baby clothing is no fun!

A portable changing pad can sometimes be nice if you need to change your baby and there is no station around.

If you travel often, a travel bassinet or pack-n-play can be extremely convenient. Not all hotels have cribs available, and if you're staying with friends without kids, they won't either.

Monitors. Again, there are a ton of options, and your personal preference will prevail here. But a good video monitor can save you so much time and energy. You can see your baby and don't have to walk to them when you hear a noise to see if they're OK, especially if they are upstairs or in some other far-off part of the home. Many times, a baby will just wake up briefly, cry out, and go back to sleep (as you'll learn in the sleep section later). There's no need to go to them when you can just check the monitor.

Don't Waste Your Money

If you're breastfeeding, you'll likely get sucked into the notion that you need an entirely new wardrobe consisting of nursing bras and nursing tops and nursing dresses. Most of them are more hassle than they're worth. You're better off purchasing a couple of simple, unpadded, nursing bras or tank tops and wearing them under baggy shirts. Once you start breastfeeding you don't want multiple layers.

I remember wearing a nursing bra (it's a bra that unhooks on the cup to allow your breast to make an easy appearance) under a nursing shirt. The shirt just had a really elastic neckline so you could pull it down easily. I was in public, so I also had my nursing scarf/apron. So, I put the apron around my neck and covered my front. I got my daughter under the apron, and with one hand I pulled my nursing top down and tried to unlatch the nursing bra. While I'm trying to do this, my squirming baby gets ahold of the apron and pulls it completely to one side so my boob is exposed. There were just too many things happening at once! Too many layers!

Later I learned that a simple nursing tank under a large or billowy shirt is ideal. Then you don't even need the cover. You discreetly unhook one strap from the nursing tank, lift up the big shirt and your baby lies across your lap and most people cannot even tell you're nursing. Your torso is still covered by the nursing tank, and the top of your boob is covered by the billowy shirt.

I do not like swings and do not recommend them. They are too often used for sleep and are not safe. I want to repeat this. Swings are not safe for newborns to sleep in and even can be dangerous for some older babies, too. I mention this in the sleep chapter, but babies should sleep on their backs on a flat, firm surface. Inclined sleepers are not safe as an infant's airway can become restricted. Also, from a sleep hygiene perspective, if you get your baby only used to sleeping in a swing or inclined seat, you likely will have trouble ever getting them to sleep in the crib.

Ahhh the SNOO. What a wonderful invention... for the first several weeks. This crib does all the things. It shushes your baby. It rocks them. It even rocks faster if they cry louder. All of these are wonderful and helpful until your baby's circadian rhythm takes over and they need a consistent nap routine. After a certain age, no amount of shushing and rocking will get your baby to sleep if they don't have a routine. I don't want to get too much into this now because I get into way more detail in the sleep chapter, but I'll just say there's a reason it's really expensive to rent a SNOO for the first few months and way cheaper after. It's just not as effective as the months go on.

Don't waste money on a ton of toys. Until your baby figures out they have hands and can use those hands as tools, your baby won't be playing with anything. If you want to spend money on something, buy books. You can read to your baby from day one!

Little tiny shoes. OMG they're so cute, but more than likely your baby will kick them off and you'll end up losing one or both of them. And, if you haven't tried, getting shoes on a baby is a chore. A method for getting them to stay on probably doesn't exist. Can you imagine, little shoes with little buckles? Velcro helps, but shoes of any form really are unnecessary until the child is at least crawling, and you can probably wait until they are starting to walk.

Build Your Baby Registry
Contribution by Lizzie Williams, Gold Coast Doulas client

Thinking about your values can help you make quicker and more impactful decisions when it comes to organizing your baby registry. People value a variety of things when it comes to their purchases. Those values may also shift over time or from purchase to purchase. Give yourself a little bit of time to center on what those values are for you. And here are few considerations:

Sustainability

Does sustainability factor into how many items you add to your list and what you choose to live without? What about the sourcing of the products? How far away are the items? What is the likelihood an item will end up in a landfill? Will you opt for new versus second-hand items?

Health

Do you want to actively avoid toxic materials, such as plastics containing BPAs? Are the items on your list best for the baby's physical development?

Baby-centered

Is it important to you to purchase items rooted in early childhood research and philosophies, such as Montessori?

Size

What can you realistically accommodate? How big is the nursery, closets, storage areas, the garage?

Aesthetics

Does beautiful design factor into your purchase decisions? Do you have a particular style you want to align with purchases?

Cost

Where does cost rank compared to your other values? Perhaps this plays a bigger role in some decisions and a smaller role in others.

Convenience

How easy would it be for guests to get the items on your list? Do they have a decent return window if you don't end up needing something, or wind up with duplicates?

Ease of use

Determining your level of comfort with complexity is important. Do you want something in a kit that requires assembly? There are many circumstances in those early days that can be typified by the dreaded notion of needing to secure nine buttons on your wiggling and irritable newborn after another overnight blowout. How much work do you want to add? You decide!

Gender preferences

If you know the gender/s of your little one, are you comfortable with particular color palettes, designs, and items often given to them based on gender or would you rather keep the colors neutral?

Shopping preferences

Are you committed to local businesses over global online retailers? Do you prefer to spend your dollars with Black-owned businesses? B-corps? Women-owned businesses? Whatever your preference, it's good to be aware of it prior to building your registry list, and realize a lot of the people shopping for you have never thought about this.

• • • •

Pets

Let's think about your fur baby. I'm sure they are perfectly well-behaved, but how will they do when a baby enters the house? Have you considered any special training for a dog? If you think your dog may have trouble adjusting to a baby, be sure to reach out to a local dog trainer who has experience with this type of training. You can do this now, while pregnant, to prepare your dog for changes in the home.

Home Organization

Your home is going to turn into baby central. You may not believe it now, but you may have a diaper changing station in your living room and bouncy seat in the bathroom or kitchen (just not on the counters or other elevated surfaces, OK?!).

What if you have a cesarean birth and can't walk up and down stairs, but the nursery is on a different floor? Where will your baby sleep? Where will you be nursing/feeding your baby? Think about all the possible locations for baby stations. Do you need more than one? If you have a guest staying with you to help out, where will they be sleeping? Is your toddler's room right next to the nursery and will guests hear the baby cry out during the night?

Think through postpartum scenarios in relation to your specific living space, and figure out what may need to change, be rearranged, or added.

Physical Recovery

Recovery looks different for everyone. Don't compare how your body or emotions recover in comparison to your best friend or your sister. If you have concerns, reach out to your health care team or a therapist.

Pelvic Floor Therapy

Until Kristin mentioned it in a previous chapter, had you ever heard of it? Your pelvic floor is a muscle but for some reason women aren't told this.

We aren't told that we can strengthen this muscle and that it's not normal to have pain during intercourse or pee while doing jumping jacks. Consider investing in pelvic floor therapy while still pregnant. Look for a trusted local pelvic floor or women's health physical therapist. This will do wonders for your ability to hold your bladder after the baby is born. It is not normal, no matter what our mothers told us, to have a weak bladder after pregnancy. Just like any other muscle in our body, if it is weak, it won't function properly. A strong pelvic floor is possible during pregnancy and after delivery.

Physical Therapy

You know your body. If you are having aches, pains, or misalignment, seek the professional care of a physical therapist. Your baby can go too! Once your baby is born, find a provider that works with babies. Physical therapists, for instance, can help your baby with torticollis, for instance. It's like a kink in the neck. It could affect your baby's ability to breastfeed because they will prefer one the side that allows them to easily turn their head. Physical therapy also can address plagiocephaly, something that many people call flat head. We see more of this than we have because of the "Back-to-Sleep" initiative. With babies safely sleeping on their backs they are more prone flattening on the back of the head. This happens simply because little baby skulls are relatively soft. Being held, worn, and being provided with tummy time during the day helps eliminate much of the flattening compared with a baby who is more regularly on their back.

Six-Week Postpartum Visit

Most moms are released to have sex and begin mild workouts at the six-week visit. Healing time is six to nine weeks on average but could be longer. Remember what we talked about earlier? Everyone's recovery time is different, so don't compare yours to anyone else's. If someone else is ready to have sex after four weeks and you aren't, that's OK.

Sex can hurt or be uncomfortable even after you are cleared. Listen to your body, and don't be afraid to ask your medical provider if you have questions or concerns. A women's health physical therapist also can be useful to eliminate or moderate painful sex.

Don't overdo it with lifting, climbing stairs, or vacuuming. Your uterus needs time to heal. You could bleed more if you overdo it. That's why having help initially is so important. Let your body rest and heal. Leave the heavy lifting to someone else for a while.

The Gross and Unexpected

Your hormones may be all over the place for a while. Plus, babies are hot, and carrying them around and nursing is hard work. You may find that you sweat. A lot. This is "extra awesome" in this stage of your life because it's really hard to find time to shower.

I want to give you a visual here. You're in the pajamas that you've been wearing for three days, no shower in days, leg and armpit hair making a comeback, and you're sweating profusely. In addition to the sweaty pits, your pajamas are covered in baby spit up, and you have spots of dried breast milk around... well, around. Your hair is up in a messy bun, not necessarily a cute one. Your hair is greasy and you're not quite sure what that brownish stuff is on the side of your neck, and you don't really care. This is what the newborn phase looks like to most, not the Insta perfect photos we see online.

As if sweating all day wasn't bad enough, you may find that you get especially hot at night. Keep your room cool. This is important for proper sleep regardless. Around 67 degrees is ideal. If you find that you have night sweats, keep water next to your bed, keep the room temp cool, and wear light layers. Waking up in a pool of sweat is no fun, plus, who has time to clean sheets?

Your Ta-Tas

Your boobs have a mind of their own whether you breastfeed or not. Most pregnant mothers will see a dramatic shift in size, sometimes during pregnancy but almost always after delivery. As your body begins to produce milk, your breasts will swell. Sometimes a little bit and sometimes a lot (whoa!). Some mothers have really tender breasts, some hurt, some find it just very uncomfortable.

My boobs got so big. Like bonkers big. As soon as my milk came in, they got tender and uncomfortable for at least a week or two until I figured out the supply and demand arrangement I had with my baby. It took a while to not always feel engorged.

You could have leaking, cracked nipples, engorged breasts, or mastitis. Find a local IBCLC to reach out to if you need help with latch, milk production, mastitis, or comfortably stopping milk production if you are ending breastfeeding.

Postpartum Bleeding

We talked about this briefly before. Postpartum bleeding, or lochia[21], is typically like a period right after you give birth. Why? Because all the stuff left over in your uterus still needs to come out. Most of it did during delivery, but there's still a bit left. Some blood and small clots are normal. If you have large clots the size of a quarter, a fever, or any other symptoms that seem alarming, reach out to your doctor. But typically, you'll just treat it like a light period and need to wear pads for a short while. It could last a couple of weeks or up to eight weeks.

First Poop

We talked about this briefly too. It's usually a scarier thought than it needs to be, but be sure to drink plenty of water, eat your greens, and take a stool softener (with approval from your doctor) if you're worried about pushing out a poo. You'll know if you need to talk to your doctor about this during pregnancy. If you're not usually regular, you generally have a hard time going, or if your bowel movements have changed while pregnant, talk to your health care team now so you can be proactive.

Gettin' Busy

Sex can be different for a while after you give birth. Remember, just because you're technically "cleared" to have sex doesn't mean you will feel ready. Talk to your partner honestly about how you are feeling, whether it's about physical pain, fatigue, or lack of desire. The physical pain should go away, and hopefully the fatigue fades soon too. Lack of desire is something you may want to speak to your doctor or therapist about. Being open and honest with your partner is critical to maintain a healthy relationship.

Hair Loss

Did you get an amazing head of hair while pregnant? Don't count on it to stick around. Those prenatal vitamins can make your skin, hair, and nails look amazing, but once baby is born your hair may start falling out. It can be alarming how much falls out or breaks off. You could also have the opposite… during pregnancy your hair and nails become dry and brittle but after baby is born they go back to normal. Everyone has a different experience with this, and as always, if there is something alarming, you should talk to your health care team about your concerns.

I never got luscious hair and nails while pregnant. My hair seemed stringy and dull and I've never had good nails. But so many of my friends and clients had amazing hair while pregnant! Many of them, even years later, tell me now that they still have spots where they feel bald because so much hair fell out after delivery.

Here are some tips on what to expect after delivery from students in our *Becoming* course and moms we polled in pregnancy groups:

"I had no idea that I would shake that much after delivery."

"I had nausea from medication and didn't expect that."

"I didn't know that I would feel cramping when the nurse pushed down on my stomach or that it would be more intense with the second baby."

"How come my friends didn't tell me how scary that first poop was after delivery?"

"I had no idea my vagina would be so swollen after giving birth."

"I didn't know recovering from a cesarean would be so difficult."

"Your second birth can be much quicker and that can be intense to process."

"I didn't know about postpartum hemorrhaging or how scary that is."

A Sense of Loss

This is something I personally didn't expect, and many of my past clients said the same thing. For months you've safely grown and housed a tiny human inside the cocoon of your uterus. You always know where they are and that they are safely tucked away inside. You are so excited to meet them, but after they're born, you may miss that baby bump. You may miss knowing that your baby is always with you, wherever you go. You may miss the ability to keep them safe and protected. It's scary out in the world.

I remember going to stroke my belly out of habit and the bump was gone. I felt really sad for a while. It was a strange feeling that I didn't expect or ever hear anyone talk about before, to feel sad that she wasn't safely inside me anymore while also being so extremely happy that she was here with me outside.

Slow Down

Embrace the necessity to slow down. Listen to your body and only do what you can and what is necessary. Leave the piles of laundry. Don't carry boxes upstairs. Don't attempt to run on the treadmill. Take it easy. Let your body heal and spend time resting and bonding with your baby. This is your time to slow down!

If you're not the type who can easily slow down, or has to always be busy, find ways to be "busy" that don't overdo it while you're healing. Maybe that's writing thank you cards, catching up on phone calls, or organizing your new baby gear.

What's important to you about your recovery? What are your goals? For instance, nutrition, getting back to exercising, making time for self-care. Keep them realistic and don't expect too much of yourself too soon. It's great to have goals but work toward them slowly.

Mood/Emotions

It's hard to explain the reality of going from a DINK (Dual Income No Kids) to motherhood, or the reality of going from one kid to two.

With your first child, one of the hardest realities is that your schedule is no longer your own. You want to run to Target real quick, you want to get your nails done, you just need to pee! Your day now revolves around this little person and it can feel like your independence is gone forever, especially if you are breastfeeding!

Life no longer seems carefree. If you were really independent before, having a baby can feel extremely restricting.

Having a second child is a huge shift. You thought caring for a newborn was hard. Now you're caring for a newborn while also trying to wrangle an on-the-go toddler. It's no longer a possibility to sleep when your baby sleeps!

No matter what situation you're in, prepare yourself for this mentally. Parenting is hard. You will have good days and bad days. Luckily, there will also be amazing days that will make up for all the bad ones.

It does get easier! With each new developmental milestone something gets easier, but oftentimes that also means something else gets harder. For instance, when your baby begins to walk. This is amazing and you think how wonderful it will be not to have to carry this little human everywhere all the time. But walking means they can go anywhere they want, and quickly! Look away for one second and they're off. This happens during the crawling stage too.

Don't be afraid or feel too proud to ask for help. It's often the only way to survive. You do not have to do this alone. If you don't have a person to physically help you in your home, reach out to friends. Find a therapist. Talk to your partner.

Baby Blues vs Depression or Anxiety

Your hormones will fluctuate drastically after you have your baby. Most mothers, four out of five[22], in fact, will experience what is known as the baby blues. This usually subsides after two weeks. You may be weepy, more emotional than is common for you, or even feel happy but still find yourself in tears. Some of what happens with baby blues may sound odd, but this is all very normal as your hormones adjust. If these feelings don't go away, though, or seem to become more serious, this is when you should take note and be more pointed about talking to someone who can help. If you're feeling extreme sadness, irritability, guilt, or having irrational thoughts, anxiety, panic attacks, or insomnia, please seek professional help. Do not wait.

And, as we've said many times, you're not in this alone. Your partner can get depressed or anxious too. This isn't all about hormones. I mentioned parenting is hard right? Lack of sleep and the emotional toll of a newborn can cause stress for partners as well. I'll say it again, ask for help! You do not need to do this alone. PMADs will be covered in detail in Chapter 11 when we discuss mental health.

Once you and your partner have knowledge of what PMADs are, there should be no guilt or shame in admitting you feel upset, angry, or scared. If you feel like you can't talk to your partner about how you are feeling, find a therapist you trust. Your doula is also a great person to talk to. Some find that verbally processing their birth with a doula or friend, and writing out their birth story while it is still fresh, can be a great exercise for healing if it is traumatic. Either way, it's great to write down as a keepsake (because you are going to forget so much so quickly).

Social Media

Don't compare yourself to Instagram moms. They're not real. What I mean is, those Instagram moms have bad days too. I promise. They just don't post pictures of themselves at 3 a.m. with poop and breastmilk all over their clothes.

Don't let your friends and family guilt you into doing something or make you feel less-than for your parenting choices. Be informed and educated so you know you're making the right decision for your family.

It's important to understand there are a wide range of emotions from pregnancy to postpartum. Some of you may have the "perfectly planned" pregnancy, birth, and postpartum experience. Others may have awful experiences, and some (if not most) will fall somewhere in the middle. Unfortunately, the negative stories are the ones that tend to circulate. The important thing is understanding there is a range, and that no matter where you fall in that spectrum, you are a good mom. No one's experience is better than another's experience. My story is different than yours but it's not better or worse, it's just mine. Comparing is harmful. Comparing creates guilt and shame, which makes it really hard for mothers to be honest with other mothers.

Having really high expectations can also be harmful. We follow the perfect Instagram Mom who had a beautiful pregnancy, all-natural delivery, her baby sleeps, breastfeeds well, Mom always looks put-together, and somehow her three-year-old is always dressed like a kid model while helping Mom make a stunningly decorated cake in their perfect kitchen. Nope.

If you think that this is reality and you set your expectations there, you are going to be very disappointed. Unless you have the funds to hire postpartum doulas around the clock, hire a cook and a cleaner, a stylist and fitness coach, this expectation is not attainable.

Expectations should be realistic. It's great to have goals and plans, but when it comes to a baby, they don't care about your goals! If you're a planner, plan to be kind to yourself. If things don't go as planned, you're still a great mother. If you have a Cesarean birth, if you don't breastfeed for as long as you wanted, if you feel overwhelmed, if you haven't showered in five days, or if you cry because you miss parts of your old life, it's OK.

These unrealistic expectations set us up for failure before we even start.

Working with so many new moms has given me an insider's view. I hear the stories of guilt, sadness, and frustration. Here are some of the most common reasons mothers have told me they think they have failed.

Using Formula

This is caused by an unrealistic expectation around breastfeeding. Mothers set an agenda for breastfeeding before they even know how much their breasts can produce or how long their baby will want to breastfeed. So, if a mother doesn't breastfeed for as long as planned, they've failed? If their baby weans naturally before the mother wanted, they've failed? If they find that they don't produce enough milk to exclusively breast-feed and have to supplement with formula, they've failed? If they decide they don't like breastfeeding, they've failed? This is all made up in their heads because of unrealistic expectations. Because they've been told, and convinced themselves, that they have to breastfeed, and do it exclusively, for a specific amount of time or else...

Or else what? What do we think will happen if our baby gets some formula? Or if our baby breastfeeds for six months instead of two years? These fears usually stem from some sort of insecurity we have way deep down, and I know I keep saying it, but a therapist can really help get to the root of where these unrealistic expectations originate.

This sense of failure can also be caused because of pressure from friends, family, and, of course, social media.

Bonding

Some mothers take to their new role immediately and bonding happens from the second they give birth. If you're a mother who doesn't feel that bond right away, this can cause you to feel extremely guilty. Please understand that bonding is different for everyone.

On the other hand, parents also have to realize that their baby may bond differently than they expect. Each baby is a unique human with unique needs and a unique personality. As your baby grows and develops, you'll notice they may bond in a different way than you anticipated. And that's fine. That's normal.

Let's say you need physical touch and lots of talking when you're upset. Does your partner have the same needs? Does your best friend? Your child will have different needs too, and that doesn't mean they aren't bonding with you. They just need something different than you. This is really important to notice and understand as early as you can because as your child gets older this will help you understand them, help them regulate their emotions, bond, and build trust.

Parenting Styles

To be or not to be…an attachment parent. That is the question.

No matter where you look, there's research telling you what you want to hear.

Babies who aren't held for the majority of the day will feel unloved.

Babies who are held all day will be spoiled.

I could go on for hours with conflicting statements like these. The only answer here is "you do you". What feels right for your family? Not your friend's family. Not your sister's, or your neighbor's, but your family.

Maybe you think that you don't want to baby wear but then you realize a few weeks in you love having your baby close, as well as being hands-free. Change your mind, that's good!

Maybe you think you want to bed-share, but you can't sleep and you're nervous about safety, so you decide to keep your baby in a bassinet near your bed. Change your mind, that's OK!

Don't get stuck in an expectation before you even know what to expect from motherhood or your baby. It's easy to let other people's opinions sway us. There's nothing wrong with saying that you're not making rules or expectations for you or your baby's experience out here until your baby arrives.

Remember we talked about how harmful unrealistic expectations can be? If you go into this with a plan, knowing you need to be flexible and open, you will be less likely to feel guilty about the decision. How can you possibly know what parenting style you will be implementing when you don't know what the temperament of your child is? Parents with more than one child will tell you that they sometimes have to parent their children differently based on that individual child's needs.

Listening, watching, and being intentional about responding to what your child needs instead of what you think they need, or what you want to give, is a huge step in learning who your child is. That, in and of itself, is your best parenting style. We get so caught up in putting labels on everything that we get stuck in "being an attachment parent no matter what" that it ends up being detrimental to our child. If attachment parenting isn't the style that works best for your kids, be open to change. If a more free-range approach is your style, but doesn't work for your child, be open to change. You may find your kid needs structure and thrives on routine (most do), but if you're too rigid your child will not have the freedom to grow either.

Alone Time

As a new mother, you won't get much alone time for a while. Wanting or needing time alone can make mothers feel guilty. For some reason we think that if we aren't 100 percent focused on our children round the clock we are bad moms.

If you need time alone it doesn't mean you don't love your child.

Personally, it took me a while to figure this out. I became resentful of my husband for going about life as normal while I was "stuck" at home all the time with a baby. He looked at me one day, gave me a hug, and said something like, "Make plans. Leave her with me. Go out with your friends. It's you that's holding yourself back." He didn't say those words exactly but that's the basic idea. In that moment I realized I was holding myself back! Why didn't I make plans or just go out? Why did I feel like I had to be there for our daughter 24/7? As she got older, I realized that I not only needed the time away for myself, but I wanted her to see that I took time away. I wanted her to know that her mom has a life outside of her; that I work, have fun with friends, and go on dates with her dad. That became really important to me. I wanted to raise a strong, independent thinker, and I didn't feel like I was doing that by staying home with her all day and revolving my entire world around her.

With that said, she still is my world! I would drop anything for her if she needed me and she knows that. But she also sees and understands that I value my time working, my time with friends, as well as my time with family.

Your parenting style can be a big factor in the amount of alone time you get but can also determine how you react to other parents' choices. An attachment parent can make others feel guilty for wanting time alone. Or I've met attachment parents who want time alone but are too embarrassed or scared to admit it because their friend circle would frown upon it.

If you want alone time, but all of your friends talk trash about mothers who hire babysitters or use a daycare provider or drop the kids off at the grandparents (consider yourself fortunate!) you're unlikely to admit that you need that.

For those of you who are not attachment parents, if you meet one that seems to love being with her kids 24/7, don't judge. Just because you can't imagine wanting that, don't assume that everyone else feels the same way as you. This is a two-way street. Do you want them to look at you and assume you neglect your children? I mentioned before that understanding others helps us to support them and empathize instead of judge them. This doesn't mean you have to fully agree with them, but being curious and supportive is a much better choice than shaming.

Parenting Can Suck

No matter what your parenting style is, it's OK to admit that parenting can suck sometimes. You will have days that you wonder why in the world you decided to do this.

Give me back my old life!

But you will also have days that make you feel a kind of joy and love you never knew you could experience. Parenting will be a roller coaster. It's normal to have bad days. It's OK, and I actually encourage you to admit that you have bad days.

Guess what...you're human and you're still a good mom!

Adoption/Fertility

I've worked with adoptive parents, or parents who struggled to conceive, who have many of the struggles we just talked about, and they suffer from some of the worst guilt I've seen.

They wanted a baby so badly and now they have one, so if they feel overwhelmed, upset, or need time alone they oftentimes tell themselves they don't deserve to be a parent. Or they don't want to complain or vent because then they would sound ungrateful. Or they feel shame for even thinking these things.

It doesn't matter how or when you conceived or adopted. You're a parent. You're going to have good and bad days. You're allowed to feel overwhelmed. If you don't have friends or family you can talk to about it without shame or guilt, find some new mom friends and, if I haven't mentioned it 100 times already, talk to a therapist.

Stay connected. Motherhood can feel isolating, so find your people. If you love exercise, find a local group of moms who exercise together. If you like to hike, listen to music, or read, find your people!

You're not perfect. None of us are. But parts of you are excellent! Focus on the things you're good at, too. Let's not dwell on all that you think you are doing wrong.

POSTNATAL STORIES

🗨 Tabetha Thomas, Kristin's former client

"Becoming a first-time mom at the age of 48, the euphoria of a baby growing inside my body and finally after years of fertility treatments and months of waiting, there is an overwhelming sense of responsibility once the baby is placed in your arms. Here is a life that I am now responsible for. A little piece of my soul that we have to protect.

"My pregnancy was high risk, so my specialist did not recommend vaginal birth and the physical healing from a C-section was minor in my mind, compared to the enormous job that lay ahead of us. Any physical pain from the surgery could be relieved with medication. I had high blood pressure, and some swelling in my legs and had to go get an ultrasound on my legs to make sure I did not have any blood clots.

"Emotional healing is the hardest to overcome. Once my baby was placed in my arms, I was healed from the exceptional longing to become a mother. But as an African American mother, emotionally, I had an enormous rush of fear of what my child would have to now experience in the world we live in today. I don't have the luxury of letting my child be just a child. She will always be a Black child or an African American child and with that understanding comes a new set of fears and constant anxiety. It is a heavy load on her that I fight on a daily basis to lift off of her shoulders.

"The bonding as a family is so natural and so loving. The immersion with family was easy. I knew she was loved from the moment we knew it was safe for me to announce my pregnancy. I waited longer than usual because of the constant fear that doctors would tell me I was having a miscarriage. My doctor told me every day that this pregnancy would not make it. I had a hematoma that bled for weeks. Babies are miracles no matter how easy or hard they come to us."

📋 Postpartum Doula Wisdom from Alyssa

Focus on you and what you need as a new mother. Make sure you eat. Make sure you're sleeping enough. Trust your instincts and ask for help.

CHAPTER 8

Feeding Options

This is not a breastfeeding chapter. I recommend taking a breastfeeding class if you plan to breastfeed or pump. This chapter will not be about your breasts, how milk is produced, or a proper latch. Instead, it is about how to prepare for breastfeeding, bottle feeding, and/or pumping. You have several feeding options, not just one.

What's Your Plan?

Most of us, during pregnancy, decide how we will feed our baby. Do you plan to exclusively breastfeed, exclusively formula feed, exclusively pump, or maybe a mixture of two or three?

It's important to note that goals for feeding often don't go as planned. Your baby may have a different agenda than you, and that's OK. I've met mothers who planned to exclusively breastfeed for one year, then realize it was too draining, mentally and physically, so they stopped after a few weeks or months. I've met mothers who planned to exclusively breastfeed but didn't love the act of breastfeeding, or their baby couldn't latch well, so they pumped and bottle fed instead. I've met mothers who thought they'd give breastfeeding a try and formula feed if necessary and ended up nursing for two years.

The point here again is it's completely fine to have goals and plans, but don't hold yourself (or your baby) to those plans. You're just setting yourself up for frustration if/when things change.

At the end of the day, as long as your baby is getting fed, that is your goal. Whether from the breast or bottle, formula, or breastmilk, we need to be sure our babies are healthy and thriving.

If you do not plan to breastfeed, prepare yourself for pushback from certain mom groups, and even certain friends and family members. Go back to the section on communication and decide how you will let people know about this decision, because they will most certainly ask. Although it's none of their business, it's wise to prepare yourself for this so you can reply confidently, without guilt or shame. You should not feel guilty for feeding your baby in whatever manner you are most comfortable.

Breastfeeding parents should take a class. It can be harder than you anticipate! For some moms it comes naturally, and they have no problems, but for most it's more difficult than we expected. Maybe your baby has a tongue tie, the latch isn't quite right, and your nipples are sore, you can't tell if you're producing enough, you get mastitis, the list goes on and on. Find a local, trusted IBCLC and have her number handy. If she offers a class or your hospital offers one, take it.

If you have a partner, doula, or other caregiver, be sure to talk to them about how they can best support you while breastfeeding. A good breastfeeding class instructor will have a section about this in her class. When you have continuous support from someone else, you are much more likely to have a more successful breastfeeding journey.

Create a nursing/feeding/changing station in a convenient spot within your home. I mentioned this in a previous chapter, but it's important to note again here because no matter how you feed your baby, you will spend a lot of time in this spot.

Think about where the station needs to be. Where do you spend the most time? You probably don't want to have to walk up or down a flight of stairs to get to your station. Maybe you set up more than one if you have different levels in your home.

Find a spot that is quiet and cozy. One where you can relax. This is important for your mindset and your letdown, which is when milk flows, if you are breastfeeding. You should look forward to entering this space, not dread it. If you like your spaces to be tidy, this is something your partner or another caregiver can help with. Keep this space clutter free, clean, and well-stocked. Amidst the chaos of the day, when you enter this space to feed your baby, make it a relaxing one. You can play soft music or light a candle. Do something that makes this space special for you and your baby since you will be in this space so often.

Scheduled Feedings vs On-Demand Feedings

This is a tough question to answer because it's so personal and varies from mother to mother and even from baby to baby. It also depends on if a mother is breastfeeding or bottle feeding, your parenting style, and the temperament of your baby. But I'll give it a go anyway because it's such a common question.

To put it simply you have two choices: feed on demand or on a schedule. In the beginning you're always feeding on demand no matter what you may want or plan for later. The first week or two especially, because your baby and you are new at this whole feeding thing, and you both just need time to figure it out. You need to figure each other out.

Your newborn will have very few needs in the beginning. A cry usually means hunger or a dirty diaper. If they are overtired, they could cry too. We will cover more of that in the sleep chapter. But a newborn typically sleeps a lot. They aren't able to stay awake very long, basically just enough to feed, then they fall back asleep. So, in the newborn phase there's not usually much crying due to tiredness and sleep.

Typically, a newborn eats every two to three hours. They will wake up, cry out, and you feed them. Pretty simple, right? Ha!

Let's say it's been a couple weeks, feeding is going well, and your baby can go about three hours between feeds. That's great! Without trying, your baby is on a schedule. You know that each of your baby's feeds, whether from the breast or a bottle, are keeping them full for approximately three hours.

Now let's say it's been four weeks, you're feeding on demand, and your baby wants to feed every 60 minutes. If you're fine with that and your baby is healthy, gaining weight, and thriving, there's no reason to change things up. If you don't like having to feed every hour you can schedule a lactation visit to see if you can increase those milk feeds so your baby can last longer stretches between each feed. If you're bottle feeding, increase the amount given in small increments to see how much your baby needs to be full.

What I'm going to say next is something I will repeat in the next chapter about sleep. Milk feeds are a very important part of a routine that is very important for optimal sleep. A hungry baby doesn't sleep well.

So, think about it this way. If your baby eats and their tummy is not full, they will cry out again in a short amount of time for another feed. This creates short windows of time for sleep, changing, playtime, and other activity in between feeds. If your baby's tummy is full, they can go longer stretches between feeds, which allows for longer stretches of time for sleep, changing, playtime, and other activities. Make sense? A longer stretch between feeds also allows you the opportunity to leave and run errands, make a call, grab a coffee, or have a quick visit with a friend.

Whether or not you schedule feeds, feed on demand, or fall somewhere in between is completely up to you. Most working parents need to have their baby on some sort of routine. Most attachment parents may feed on demand as they will likely be holding or wearing their baby the majority of the day. Remember, your lifestyle, parenting style, and finally your baby's temperament will determine these decisions.

OK, back to feeding. Keeping in mind that your newborn will need to feed every two to three hours, you must realize that this means 24/7. They don't just feed every two to three hours during the day; they do all night long, too. If your newborn doesn't wake up to eat, wake them! It's crucial they wake to eat when they are this young. If your newborn is too sleepy to wake up, and you are struggling to get them to feed, reach out to your pediatrician. Don't celebrate because you have a "good sleeper". All healthy newborns sleep a lot, but they need to feed often too. They need the calories and nutrients to gain weight.

If you're unsure, ask your pediatrician or your lactation consultant. They can weigh your baby and will tell you if they have any concerns. You want to make sure your baby is gaining weight and thriving.

On the other hand, if you have a baby that doesn't seem to be able to sleep much, talk to your pediatrician about that, too. Your newborn should basically sleep and eat all day and all night, waking only to eat and give you short minutes of awake time before or after feeding. Remember that a hungry baby won't sleep very long, so be sure to eliminate that as a possibility right away.

For a mother who bottle feeds, whether it's formula or breastmilk, you may get longer stretches between feeds right away. This is because you have a visual of how much your baby is actually eating. Most exclusively breastfeeding mothers wonder how much their baby is getting. For a mother who exclusively breastfeeds, the length of time between feeds will really depend on how much milk you produce and how efficient your baby is at draining your breast. If you have a baby that wants to "snack" all day long every hour, they aren't getting one full feed. After two to three weeks of figuring out this feeding situation with your baby, you should start to see a feeding pattern form. After a few weeks, a baby getting full feeds can usually go two to three hours between feeds.

As your baby grows, they become stronger, and they develop muscles in their jaw to feed more efficiently. Take note that some changes will occur. If you are bottle feeding, there are different nipple sizes and different flow levels. A newborn nipple will have a very small hole and the milk or formula will come out slowly. As your baby gets stronger, they can handle a faster flow. Check the bottle and/or nipple you are using to make sure you're graduating to different levels as your baby grows. For a breastfed baby, a full feeding session that used to take 40 minutes now may only take 25. This doesn't mean your baby is getting less milk, they are just getting better at eating.

I remember a sleep client of mine once telling me she was really worried about her baby's feeds because they had been happening so quickly the past couple months. The baby could go four hours between feeds but she was trying to feed him earlier assuming he must be hungry since his last feed only took 20 minutes and they used to take well over 30. I had to remind her that her 5-month-old was much bigger and stronger than he was at three and four months. He is healthy and happy and can go four hours between feeds. He was getting all the calories he needed in a shorter amount of time.

You will have to decide if you want to be an on-demand feeder or feed on a schedule, keeping in mind that schedules always have to be flexible. You can't hold a newborn to a schedule and watch the clock. By schedule I mean "my baby can go about three hours between feeds." That's a loose schedule. If your baby cries from hunger after 2 ½ hours, you aren't going to watch the clock for 30 minutes and let them cry so you can feed them in exactly three hours. With that said though, this is where a pacifier comes in handy. This is what it's supposed to be used for, to temporarily pacify your baby. In this instance, you would use the pacifier until you can feed them. Let's say you're 10 minutes away from home, or on a walk. You can give your baby a pacifier until you can get home to feed them.

If you have a baby that wants to feed on-demand all day every hour and you love it, then, as I mentioned, keep doing it! Don't let anyone else tell you it's wrong. If your lifestyle doesn't allow for that, then work on bigger feeds during the day so your baby can go longer between each feed. As long as your baby is growing, gaining weight, and thriving per your pediatrician, your feeding routine is fine, no matter what you choose.

If you want to try and increase feeds for your little snacker, try this. If your baby snacks at the breast for five minutes and falls asleep, and then 30 minutes later snacks for five minutes, and an hour later for another five minutes, try to increase those 5-minute snacks to 10-minute feeds. That might mean feeding in a well-lit area, removing layers so they aren't so warm and cozy, or tickling them to keep them awake. See how long your baby can go in-between each feed now. Then, what happens if you increase those feeds to 15 minutes? That could be the difference between a snack and meal for a baby. For bottle fed babies, like I mentioned before, increase by small increments, and see how long you can go between feeds.

If you decide to breastfeed it could be beneficial for you to find some breastfeeding groups to join, whether locally or online. La Leche

League is a popular one, support groups (Facebook, hospitals, lactation consultants sometimes have their own, doula agencies), and postpartum support groups.

Certified Lactation Consultants (IBCLCs and CLCs) are so important to your breastfeeding journey if you find you're struggling. And I want to tell you they don't just help you with a proper latch and increasing milk production. They help if you don't want to breastfeed and want to minimize pain and discomfort while your milk comes in. They help with weaning, pumping, and some even with bottle feeding.

You'll probably see one or many lactation consultants in the hospital and they may or may not be helpful. Many of my clients had a dreadful time with breastfeeding and/or the lactation consultant in the hospital but ended up figuring things out when they got home or hired an in-home IBCLC to visit. Find out if any in your area do in-home consults, and don't forget to check with your insurance provider ahead of time and see what's covered. You may find out that lactation classes or visits are covered.

Breastfeeding can be isolating. Newborns eat a lot, and you can feel like that's all you do… all day long. As your baby grows, remember you should start to notice a feeding pattern. Even if you don't want a set schedule, try to have a routine. This not only helps you plan your day, but kids thrive on routine.

For instance, let's say your baby is up for the day at 7 a.m. and feeds. You know your baby will stay awake for about 30 minutes after the feed, because that is what you noticed they've been able to do before needing a nap again. Repeat this several times throughout the day, then have them go to bed at 7 p.m. That is a very loose routine, but with a set wake time and bedtime. This is great for parents who don't want a strict schedule. They still follow their baby's cues all day, and then have a relatively reliable wake time and bedtime.

Pumping

If you have maternity leave and plan on returning to work, you'll need to think about pumping if you're breastfeeding. If you're not breastfeeding, you will have already figured out how many bottles of formula your baby needs during the day while you're gone.

For breastfeeding mothers, you will want to test out your pump a couple weeks before you're due back at work. If breastfeeding is going well, there's no need to get that pump out prior. I say this because I've seen so many moms get caught up with nursing and pumping and storing milk that they drive themselves mad. Not only do they have no free time, but it becomes this strange competition with themselves to see how much they can get in the freezer.

With that said, there may be a couple reasons why you'd want to get the pump out earlier. Maybe your lactation consultant or pediatrician told you to pump because they are concerned about milk supply. Maybe you are exhausted and want your partner or your doula to feed the baby in the night, so you pump and they bottle feed. Maybe you are ready for your first outing and you need to pump and leave a bottle for someone to feed the baby while you're gone.

If you've never used a breast pump before, prepare yourself for some giggles. It's a pretty strange sensation to put plastic flanges over your nipples, turn a machine on that starts sucking them in and out, and then watch milk fill bottles like a cow at the farm. They're noisy, not the most comfortable, and just look ridiculous.

An important thing to note about breast pumps is that there are different flange sizes so make sure yours fit properly. This depends on your nipple size so look up your pump and how the flange is supposed to fit. You don't want it too small or too large. Both of these scenarios will cause pain. You can also ask your lactation consultant which flange size is best for you.

When you pull out your pump a couple weeks before going back to work, this is when you can start working on a small supply of milk for your freezer. No need to overdo it. It's always reassuring for a mother to know there's a little extra in the freezer, but each day at work you'll be pumping what you need for your baby the following day. So, if you've been told you need a stockpile, that's not true. Think about all the time it will take for you to create the stockpile. If you have the extra time, go for it! But most mothers are too tired, so just pump an extra few ounces here and there if you want.

To put pumping at work into perspective, you'll wake up on Monday for work. Depending on what time you have to get there, you may have time to nurse your baby before you go. If not, you can pump and leave a bottle for the caregiver to feed once it's baby's wake time. Let's say your baby eats every three hours. Depending on how many hours you will be at work, you may need to pump two or three times. What you pump on Monday will be what your baby eats on Tuesday while you're at work. You will have to figure out what milk you use on Monday. It's usually easiest to save Friday's pumped milk in the fridge and use that the following Monday. Over the weekend, you'll be feeding from the breast. Obviously, if you have weekend plans, just pump a bottle for the babysitter or caregiver before you leave.

Does your workplace have a pumping room? Does your state require it? How will you fit pumping breaks into your workday? Ask your employer your questions before you go back to work. Ideally you can have this all figured out while you're pregnant and still at work.

If you are nervous about pumping, or if you find it's harder than you expected, consider a pumping class before returning to work. Some lactation consultants offer them, and if not, they may offer an in-home pumping consultation.

Multiples

You think feeding one baby is tough, try feeding two or three at once! If you're having multiples, it's important to have help in your home those initial weeks. With twins or triplets, having a set of hands for each baby is really helpful. Think ahead about what kind of help you may need later. Get support lined up. Find a postpartum doula that is skilled with multiples. Have friends and family members take shifts. Can anyone stay overnight?

Having your babies on a consistent feeding schedule will be critical. Having multiples is one scenario where feeding on demand isn't an option. You will run yourself ragged.

If you're nursing multiples, feed one at the breast and have someone else feed the other(s) with a bottle at the same time. Then, for the next feed, feed the other one at the breast, and the other(s) with a bottle. That way your breasts will be an equal opportunity employer. We want all babies to have equal time at the breast.

If you don't have help at home, you may find it's easier to pump and bottle feed both babies at the same time. You may also get the hang of nursing one while bottle feeding the other. Nursing two at a time can be difficult, but an IBCLC can help with nursing multiples if that is a goal. Give yourself time to figure out which feeding strategies work best for you, how well your babies are eating, and try to allow yourself some breaks.

Eventually, you'll probably get used to feeding two or three at a time and once the babies can hold their own bottles it gets much easier. I took a multiples training several years ago and there was a section about becoming an octopus. With multiples you will literally feel like one! You'll be holding babies and bottles and burp cloths using both hands, your feet, your shoulders, and the crooks of your arms and legs. Mothers of multiples display multitasking at its finest.

Bonding

Sometimes mothers have this notion that breastfeeding is going to create an amazing bonding experience with their baby, and for many that's true. But remember when we talked about having empathy for mothers, especially those mothers who may be suffering from a PMAD? Feeding can be a source of anxiety and depression for some. Sometimes this stems from past sexual trauma. They may feel like they expected to feel a certain way, to enjoy their newborn, to feel connected to their baby, and they feel guilty admitting that they aren't. They feel guilty because they aren't bonding like they imagined and because breastfeeding is hard or uncomfortable or they want to formula feed. If you are a mother who bonded right away and loved breastfeeding, please be aware that there are mothers who decide to stop or who may admit to you that they're having a rough time. They need your support, not your judgment.

Bonding is not always instant for everyone, and it can happen in many ways at different stages of motherhood. I've heard some mothers express that they feel connected to their baby while breastfeeding or bed sharing, while others say they feel most bonded while snuggling their well-rested baby after a night of sleep alone. Others feel the most bonded during a bedtime routine while they snuggle and sing to their baby. While others bond during awake moments with play and laughter. Many partners feel a bond while bottle feeding. Bonding looks different for everyone because we all have such different styles, personalities, goals, and families. That means that yes, even a bottle-feeding parent can have amazing bonding experiences with their baby! Babywearing can be great. Reading and singing to your baby are wonderful. Find what works best for you. Just because someone else bonds with their baby one way doesn't mean it's the right way for you.

If breastfeeding isn't the amazing bonding experience you expected, or you find that it is affecting your mental health, call an IBCLC, a therapist, or talk to your doula or medical provider. Figure out what your best solution is. Exclusively pumping? Formula feeding? The most important point here is to admit that you're struggling and ask for help. No matter what, we need to make sure your baby is properly fed.

Older Siblings

Bringing home, a new baby can be a hard transition for an older sibling depending on the age. Do you have a two-year-old who tends to hit? Or a three-year-old who is jealous of the new baby taking you away from him? It will be very important to find ways to make the older sibling understand that they are loved and are special, particularly while you feed the baby and during other tasks that take so much time.

One-on-one time with your older child will be so important. Until now they've been your one and only. They got you to themselves. Now this newer, smaller creature has entered their home and taken over. You know your child best. How could you help them understand that they are loved?

The bedtime routine often is a great time to focus on some one-on-one. If they don't already have a set bedtime and a routine, you may want to start working on this now while you're still pregnant. We will talk more about the importance of a bedtime routine in the next chapter, but having a special routine for this child, no matter what, will help create an independent experience that conveys love and attention and amid the chaos of a newborn.

You may have to get creative for times like feeding when you must focus solely on the baby. You can make feedings at a time when your older child gets to do something they like. Maybe it's watching a show or playing with toys from a special bin that they only get to play with at feeding time. Make it age-appropriate for your child.

For older kids, giving them age-appropriate responsibilities can help them feel like a big kid. When you ask them to help with the baby it makes them understand that they can do all sorts of awesome things that the baby can't. They may need to feel smarter, bigger, or think they are more important to help negate feelings of jealousy.

Breastfeeding tips from an RN, IBCLC

Kelly Wysocki-Emery, MSN, RN, IBCLC is a breastfeeding educator for Gold Coast Doulas and the owner of Baby Beloved, Inc. Kelly has been helping mothers breastfeed since 1994. She works in private practice as well as for a hospital system, and splits her time between the hospital, six pediatric offices, and private home consultations. She also teaches breastfeeding classes through Gold Coast as well as virtually and in-person through Baby beloved, Inc, which she loves. Kelly breastfed two babies, and it was those babies who changed her trajectory in life to become a lactation consultant.

Most everyone has a common-sense knowledge that breastfeeding is best for infants and mothers, from a nutritional, immunological, and a bonding standpoint. Most women these days start out breastfeeding, and halt the practice, for various reasons, prior to what was intended. Some do not have easy access to lactation consultants, some do not have the support of their family or doctor, and some just hit a wall and say "no more" for their own reasons. When we become a mother, we don't do so in a vacuum. We bring all our own preferences, needs, and personality into the mix, as well as outside commitments (like a job, or work, school, caring for a sick family member) and our relationships (our friends, husband/partner, our own mother). The culture you happen to be born into weighs into our breastfeeding choices and behaviors, so each woman and partner will look at breastfeeding in a unique way.

So how do you stack the odds in your favor?

I like to remind women in my breastfeeding class that their grandmother and great-grandmother, and every other female before her, probably did not take a breastfeeding class. They had "on the job" training from their baby and their many sisters/cousins/aunts/friends who were in constant contact with her after the baby came. Don't get me wrong, education about our bodies is never a bad thing, and never wasted time, but if our ancestors have been able to do this since time began, we can probably figure things out as well. My intention by bringing this up is not to be glib, but to help women connect to their amazing, miraculous, strong mammalian lineage. This inherited gift is for all women to claim, but it can take time to be comfortable with nursing, even though it is a "natural" thing. Sex is a natural thing, too, but think how awkward it was the first time you engaged in it. As with anything, it takes time to find your groove and feel confident.

Breastfeeding is an elaborate dance, and each mother will need to take the time to figure out what works for both of them. Offer yourself and your baby a ton of grace as you are getting to know each other through your breastfeeding experience. Think of the first day on the job. Did you know how to do everything confidently from day one, without mistakes or questions? Probably not. Only with coming to work each day, asking for help and mentorship from your boss and co-workers, were you able to hit your stride.

This holds true for breastfeeding. I highly recommend going to a support group both before and after having the baby to ask your questions, listen to other women's stories, and to watch how breastfeeding happens in real life. Being around other women is, I think, how women have traditionally gotten through their breastfeeding challenges. We are not meant to be in isolation when it comes to motherhood. Finding your breastfeeding buddies will go a long way toward helping you learn how to breastfeed with confidence.

The Breast Crawl

Your baby has been hardwired to do something called the "breast crawl". This is when baby is placed on mother's chest and abdomen immediately after delivery and the baby is given time to scoot/crawl/throw themselves over to the breast and latch on all by themselves. It is the most incredible thing to witness.

When I first started encouraging mothers to do this, it was very difficult for me to not reach in and help latch on baby. I literally had to, and sometimes still do, put my hands behind my back so I stay out of the magic. Without help from the "experts", human mammals, like every other mammal on the planet, can find their way to the breast through their various instincts. Humans have over 20 instincts that help them crawl to the breast when left alone. It usually takes about 30 to 60 minutes after delivery before baby starts the trek, and they usually can make it. I believe this takes a little pressure off the mother, from feeling as though she has to do all the work and that her latching skills have to be perfect. No other mammal on the planet latches their young. Our babies are smarter than we realize and can amaze you with their mad skills if you let them. And if you have a Cesarean section, or if mother or baby need medical attention right after delivery, no worries—these instincts are in place for a long time, and you can try it out once everyone is settled and ready, hours or even days after the baby is born.

Whether you breastfeed or bottle-feed pumped milk and/or formula, know that your love will undoubtedly flow through to your baby. Yes, breastfeeding is the ideal nourishment for babies, but even more important is the relationship you have with feeding your baby. I know that may sound odd coming from a lactation consultant who has spent her entire career trying to help mothers breastfeed their babies, but there are times when the effort interferes with the mother's mental health and her relationship with her baby, and at that point, the mother-infant relationship is more important than the breastmilk. This will be a very personal decision for each mother, and her feelings about breastfeeding may change from time to time, and this is very normal.

If breastfeeding is not turning out the way you hoped it would, I want to let you in on a little secret. It doesn't have to be an "all or nothing" situation. If you need to use formula, that doesn't mean you cannot still put your baby to your breast for warmth, bonding, and comfort (and even a partial amount of breastmilk). I encourage mothers who are struggling with their decision on whether to stop nursing to consider holding on to the things they DO love about breastfeeding for as long as desirable. For instance, nursing baby after a partial bottle is a lovely way to offer baby "dessert at the breast". Baby will be calm, snuggly, and still getting some of your sweet, lovely milk.

A Partner's Role

I always like to take the opportunity to let the baby's other parent know that their support can mean the difference in breastfeeding success. No pressure, but research shows that the support, attitude, and practical help a partner offers to the breastfeeding parent bears more weight than what the doctors, nurses, or even the lactation consultants have to say. They love this baby as much as the nursing parent does, and they will be there at 2 a.m., and they will know what words to say to encourage you if the going gets rough.

Having a partner on board for the breastfeeding journey is highly recommended, and if they will come to a breastfeeding class to help gather the information, all the better. Four ears are better than two. Some advice I give to the other parent is to ask the nursing parent what they need. What foods they like. What pillows would be helpful. Can I burp the baby or change her diaper now? Be the gatekeeper to unwelcome visitors. There are plenty of ways to participate in breastfeeding without breasts, and those gestures are more important than you may imagine.

What Breastfeeding May Look Like

Not everyone wishes to put the baby directly to the breast, for whatever their personal reasons. Pumping and bottle feeding these days is a much more viable option as the technology (and the Affordable Care Act) have made it easy to get a quality pump that can maintain a good milk supply in place of a latching baby. As more mothers are breastfeeding, the market has ended wildly with products that help make pumping more convenient. Products such as a pumping bra allow you to pump while having your hands free to eat lunch, bottle-feed baby, work on your computer, read a magazine, or do breast compression to yield more milk. With a good routine and a quality pump, maintaining a milk supply with a breast pump can be an option.

If you are returning to work or school, having a conversation with your boss or instructor can help put into place a plan to support your efforts of pumping while separated from baby. According to the Pregnant

Workers Fairness Act, effective on June 27, 2023, mothers who work for a company with at least 15 employees and are paid an hourly rate or salary are allowed reasonable breaks, usually three 15- to 20-minute breaks in an eight-hour shift, to pump in a place that is private and not a bathroom. This law extends for the first two years of an infant's life, thanks to the PUMP Act that passed in 2022.

BREASTFEEDING STORIES

💬 A Breastfeeding Story from Kristin

"I ended up needing the support of lactation consultants after each birth for completely different reasons. My daughter was in the NICU for glucose issues. She started on an IV and later moved to an enhanced formula while I pumped. I was eventually able to give her my pumped milk and attempted to nurse her. When she came home from the NICU, she preferred the bottle to the breast. I was still pumping but wanted to fully transition to breastfeeding. I saw lactation consultants at the hospital and at home. I was finally able to get my daughter to latch after a lactation consultant suggested the breast crawl.

"My son was an eager eater, but I knew something was off. I mentioned the pain with nursing to my pediatrician and she noticed that my son had a tongue tie. I got that revised and things were so much better with the help of my lactation consultant. I later ended up getting thrush and mastitis and worked with my lactation consultant to overcome those issues, as well."

💬 A Breastfeeding Story from Alyssa

"I remember feeding my daughter right away as a newborn and I thought it was going so smoothly. Until I noticed my left nipple was becoming sore. Then cracked. Then bleeding. One afternoon I was sitting in the nursery sobbing, because the pain was unbearable, when my husband walked in. He took one shocked look at my nipple, turned around, and got my pump from the other room. It was still boxed, and neither of us knew how to use it, but he proceeded to unpack it and read the instructions. He said to me, 'It has to hurt less than her mouth, right?' So, I gave it a try, and yes, it did help. I got through it, but I so wish I had known I could get a lactation consultant over to my house to help me. As a first-time mom with no females in my family to guide me, I had no previous experiences to turn to. I'm also the type of person who gets things done her own, but looking back I wish I had sought help from mom and friends when I needed it."

💬 Pumping Story from Lizzie Williams, Gold Coast postpartum client and *Becoming A Mother* student

"Navigating the world as a pumping mother was one of the most eye-opening experiences of parenthood for me. I am grateful to work for a company that has an intentionally designed mother's room with a couch, refrigerator, extra breast pads, wipes, and other thoughtful touches. What I quickly realized when I began pumping is that much of the rest of the world is not as accommodating.

"One day, shortly after returning to work, I was invited to attend a team offsite on a pontoon boat. Pre-baby, this would have sounded like a dream. An afternoon hanging out with my colleagues, soaking up the sun, and sipping a seltzer or two? Awesome. As a breastfeeding mama on a strict three-hour pumping schedule, at the very best, it sounded awkward. However, I still wanted to feel like an engaged teammate, so I packed up my portable pump, a milk cooler and ice packs, a plastic bag with my clean pump-parts and extras for the dirty ones. I put on my sunscreen. My plan was to pump in the bathroom at the restaurant we were eating at prior to departure and then cross my fingers that we'd be done with the boat ride in less than three hours. As soon as I sat on the grimy restroom toilet to pump, I realized my portable pump was out of batteries. "No worries," I thought, "I'm a prepared mama! I brought the cord, just in case!" That would have been great, except there were no plugs near any of the stalls, nor was there a lock on the door. I had to shift gears fast because my team was getting ready to head to the boat. I ended up running back to my car, plugging the pump into the charger in the backseat and covering myself with a towel so passersby wouldn't see. I was so stressed out by it all that the thought of potentially getting stuck having to plug the pump into an open pontoon boat, surrounded by coworkers was too much.

"I finished pumping and simply told my team I needed to sit this one out. I share this story not to scare anyone, but just to remind you of three things: charge those batteries, be prepared for something to go awry, and give yourself permission to say no to things that are going to add stress to your life. I had to tell myself on multiple occasions, 'This is just a season', to remind myself that it's OK to make different decisions during different phases of life. There will be more boat rides."

📋 Doula Wisdom from Kristin

If you plan to breastfeed, take a breastfeeding class during pregnancy. It makes all the difference. Have your partner attend so they know how to support you as well.

📋 Postpartum Wisdom from Alyssa

If you have a postpartum doula, a family member, or friend staying with you overnight, have them sleep in the nursery with the baby, or in another room as long as it's away from you. You can get optimal sleep knowing baby is cared for while someone else wakes up with them. If you are breastfeeding, you can wake when your breasts feel full. Set an alarm for when your baby would eat next, pump, and set the pumped bottles of milk outside your door. You can go right back to sleep while the doula or other caregiver feeds your baby.

CHAPTER 9

Caring for Your Baby

Before We Get Into It

Babies cry. There's no way around it, but there are ways to minimize crying and also to learn to listen better and respond according to what you feel your baby desires. This is a skill and can be learned. Most of you, especially if you don't have a bunch of experience with kids, will not immediately understand babies' general cues and varying cries.

First, you need to figure out what works best for your baby. We know your baby will cry often for very basic needs—food, sleep, or a clean diaper. As they grow and develop, their cries communicate more, frustration, boredom, overstimulation, pain, confusion. Learn to really watch and listen.

This will be trial and error for a while. Don't assume every cry means food. This is a common mistake. If you do make this assumption, it may lead to a loop of constant feeds.

What is your baby telling you?

Find out what causes the crying and react accordingly. This could mean putting a warmer outfit on your baby because they are cold, removing a layer because they feel hot, moving their play mat over because the sun is directly in their eyes, or scheduling a doctor's visit because they seem to be in pain or frequently have a fever.

This is also the first way to instill trust between you and your baby.

Your baby will learn that you are responding to their actual needs, not just always offering food or picking them up because you think that's what they want. If I came over to your house and stubbed my toe and it started bleeding, would you offer me some fries? Or what if my daughter asked me for help with her math homework and I replied, "OK, I'll start dinner!" She would think I wasn't listening. Eventually, if I responded this way again and again, she would stop asking me for help because she wouldn't trust me. She would know I'm not paying attention to her needs.

Realize that sometimes your baby will just fuss. It may not mean anything, so leave them be. Some babies grunt and groan. Some cry out occasionally. Some babies sound like little goats, especially when they sleep. Every peep they make isn't necessarily a cry for help. Listening is a skill. Start listening early and it will be so much easier to communicate with them as your child gets older.

How Babies Communicate, and Ways to Respond

Soothing

Read Harvey Karp's *The Happiest Baby on the Block*. You will learn several ways to soothe a baby and figure out which one is best for your baby. You may find it takes several of the methods he talks about to soothe your baby.

For our purposes, the easiest way to do this is to describe what you're likely to confront based on the baby's condition. There are a bunch of common ailments that may upset your baby. Some of them you've heard of but others are things most of my clients knew nothing about until they had their babies. Let's talk about a few of them.

Diapers

Something as simple as a dirty diaper may cause your baby to cry. Stay on top of changing diapers to avoid diaper rash. This can become painful. No matter what kind of diaper you use, consider a barrier cream or butt balm. Anything that keeps moisture away from your baby's skin will help, and make sure baby's bum is completely dry before putting on a new diaper.

Reflux/Colic

This condition can make a baby very uncomfortable, and they will cry a lot. Sleep may be very disrupted, which compounds the problem. Talk to your pediatrician. Many times, babies will outgrow this in a couple months as they develop and mature.

Skin Rashes

Talk to your child's pediatrician if your baby has bad rashes. This could be the first sign of a food allergy. Regardless, a rash can get itchy and very uncomfortable. Note that some strange skin conditions are common, such as baby acne or milia. These go away on their own with time.

Another common skin condition is cradle cap. It can look like large chunks of skin peeling off your baby's head. Monitor it and reach out to your pediatrician as needed.

Teething

Some babies seem to breeze through new teeth just fine and others tend to experience more pain. You can talk to your pediatrician if you have concerns. Just know this is a temporary development that you'll be through soon.

Constipation

Most babies will eat, poop, eat, poop, eat, poop. Going days in between can be common, but if it's accompanied by any other symptoms including fever, call your pediatrician. Also, if your baby hasn't pooped in two days, prepare for a blowout when they do.

Now you can see why we can't just offer food every time a baby cries.

If they are tired, they may suck for a couple seconds then fall asleep. If they have reflux, food may actually make them more upset. If they are constipated or in pain, you may see them arching their back and avoiding food. If they have a rash, they may cry from pain or discomfort. Watch closely, especially as they get older. They are communicating with you!

Self-Care

I debated whether to put this topic here or with mood/emotions. Ultimately, I put it here because soothing a baby can seem impossible when you're not able to care for yourself.

Whatever self-care means for you, try to make it a priority, and tell your partner it's a priority. Just as you need to figure out how to best soothe your baby, communicate how your friends and family can "soothe" you.

Do you need 30 minutes alone in the morning to drink coffee and check emails? Maybe it's a shower, or a walk around the neighborhood with a friend. What do you need to feel like you? Sometimes self-care just means having difficult conversations, setting boundaries, and standing up for yourself.

Try not to get caught up in data entry (unless required for a NICU baby). If you're nursing, and pumping, and collecting data, and doing all the other things necessary to get through your day, you will run out of energy quickly. Try your best to relax and enjoy this time. Ask for help or get back to the details later.

Your Baby's Unique Personality

I want to focus on your baby's temperament for a minute. Some parents get so caught up in their goals, including their goal for a parenting style, that they fail to notice that it's not working for their baby. For instance, some babies like time to themselves. I'm not talking about the newborn stage, here, I'm talking about your baby once they are say four months or more. I've seen it so many times where a baby is content, sitting in a bouncy seat, looking at a toy or out the window, and then a visitor comes over to them, or even a caregiver or parent, and the baby resists. Even though the baby resists, the well-meaning adult proceeds. The once happy, content baby is now upset and crying. If this happens frequently, your baby may prefer quiet time. You will have to figure out what method soothes your baby best. Holding and bouncing may not be it. They may prefer to lie alone in their crib with the sound machine on or be held in your arms while you read. Parents who expect a certain soothing method to work for all babies become disappointed when it doesn't work for theirs. It can make them feel like they are doing something wrong or that there is something wrong with their baby. Or worse, that their baby doesn't like them. When in fact, if they would take a step back and realize what their baby is communicating, they can switch gears and try a different method.

For babies with this temperament, it can be difficult for attachment parents who want to hold their baby most of the time. Remember, there are so many other ways to bond and form healthy attachments with your baby. Follow their lead!

If you learn to listen and follow your baby's cues, it will be easy to carry this over into the toddler years. When your child can talk, it's so much easier, of course. But when they are crying, or asking for something, or throwing a fit, if they know you are listening and they can trust you, it makes these scenarios go so much smoother. The toddler that knows you will play with them after you finish emails will gladly wait a few more minutes because they trust you. You've proven before that you listen and follow through on your promises. The toddler who knows they can't ask for more stories at bedtime won't argue because you've already set the limit and are consistent.

As your child grows, so should their level of trust. They are smarter than you think and you can't pull a fast one on them without losing some trust. Listen to what they're asking and respond accordingly. Do what you say you will. Be consistent.

NEWBORN STORIES

💬 Newborn Stories from Dr. Rachel Babbitt, Gold Coast client and co-owner of Rise Wellness Chiropractic

"I had no idea that at my 20-week ultrasound I was going to tell me that I was having twin girls. From that moment on everything changed. The amount of doctor appointments I had increased. Suddenly I needed to buy two of everything. My plan of having a home birth suddenly changed to an induction in the hospital. Right from the start I was beginning to see that life with twins is very different. It is fun, crazy, chaotic, and super rewarding, like all babies are, just times two.

"I had a hard time asking for help at first but was very fortunate that I had a supportive husband and family. Everyone jumped in and really helped in those first few weeks of postpartum fog. With all the help in place, I eventually came to the realization that I needed and wanted to learn how to be a twin mom on my own. I slowly gained the confidence of taking care of two babies on my own. The days could be long and exhausting, but eventually I found a rhythm and schedule that worked for us. The newborn phase of life definitely looked a little different than what I imagined it would be.

"I had envisioned myself doing all the different mom group things, such as music classes, mom baby yoga, and mom meet ups. I soon realized I didn't feel comfortable or confident doing these things alone with two babies. I slowly figured out my limits. For instance, I couldn't bring both babies to the grocery store alone, but I could put them in the car and drive to visit a friend and be able to hang out with them and also have help with the twins. Knowing I had someone else to help me when I got there made all the difference.

"I am grateful that I used Gold Coast Doulas during my pregnancy because this is how I learned about what a postpartum doula was and how they could help. Once I found my footing, I used a postpartum doula to help focus on some me time and to help me feel 'normal' for a minute. They would come over and take care of the babies and I was able to shower, nap, or work out. Just having a few hours a week to have some time for myself helped me to be a more attentive and clear-headed mom. Being a twin mom becomes a way of life and I can't imagine my world without my twinners in it!"

📋 Postpartum Doula Wisdom from Alyssa

You don't need to give your baby or child a bath every day. For some reason parents are under the impression that it has to be done daily, but unless your baby has a blow-out, has dried spit up in their neck rolls, or is smelly, they probably only need a bath a couple times a week. Same with your toddler. Bathing every day can dry out skin and cause skin rashes to worsen. It is also very time-consuming for you as parents.

CHAPTER 10

All about
the ZZZZZs

I know, I know…I'm a sleep consultant so you're expecting this chapter to tell you exactly how to get your baby to sleep through the night, right? Sorry.

My sleep consultations are customized, and change based on each family, so it's impossible to tell you exactly how I can help your particular baby sleep. If I could, I would just write that book and everyone would be happy! BOOM!

But alas, I cannot. What I can do is give you some tried and true tips and tricks to work on and give you a basic knowledge of sleep so you know what's happening with your baby throughout different stages.

Deal?

Sleep Deprivation

This is the real haze of new motherhood. Remember, I mentioned that newborns eat a lot, every two to three hours. That means you're only getting sleep in small intervals. For instance, your baby feeds at 10 p.m. and takes 30 minutes to eat, then you change their diaper and put them back to sleep. So maybe, if you're lucky, by 10:45 you're back in bed. Baby will likely need to eat again at midnight or 1 a.m. Assuming you are able to fall asleep the instant your head hits the pillow, you might get one to two hours of sleep before you're at it again.

Sleep and Mental Health

Sleep deprivation is a major driver of mental illness. It was used as a torture method for a reason. Losing just two hours of sleep at night puts you in a state of impairment, worse[23] than a drunk driver. That's how important sleep is to our physical and mental well-being.

Be very careful about leaving your house, driving, and walking up and down steps with your baby if you are sleep deprived. We get clumsy and more prone to accidents when we are tired. It's always a better option to put your baby down safely in the crib or a bouncy seat if you feel like you are unwell. Even if your baby is crying, place them somewhere safe while you do what you need to do.

The inability to fall asleep can be a symptom of a PMAD but can also be a driver. If you find that even when you lie down to sleep you are unable, please talk to your health care provider or therapist right away.

We get so focused on how our babies are sleeping that we forget about our own sleep needs. Your sleep is important too. Make it a priority. Try to keep track of how many hours of sleep a night you are getting. If it's less than six or seven in those early weeks, nap when your baby is sleeping and don't allow visitors. Remember that communication chapter? Figure out ways you can gently talk to visitors about what you need. Your partner should help.

Once your baby is on a better routine, strive for a full eight hours of sleep per night. Find a reputable sleep consultant; locally if you want an in-person consult, or virtually. If you've never needed eight hours, then try to get back to as much sleep as you had before your baby. If seven hours is your jam, stick with that. Just like kids, adults have different sleep needs too. Most adults[24] need seven to eight hours per night with a very small percentage of people needing less than that.

Are there postpartum doulas in your area who offer overnight support? This is a great gift option, and an amazing way to get more rest at night those initial weeks postpartum.

Sleep Hygiene

I mentioned before that newborns sleep a lot. They will literally eat, sleep, poop, repeat. The first few weeks they won't be able to stay awake for very long at all. Let's say your one-week-old is eating every two hours. That's 12 feeds a day. If each feed takes 30 minutes, that's 6 hours of their day with the remaining 18 for sleep. That's pretty normal.

As your baby gets older, you'll notice they can stay awake for longer and longer stretches between feeds. They will also become more efficient at eating, and you'll notice they can go longer between feeds and the amount of time they need to get a full meal may decrease. When your baby can go three hours between feeds, this brings your number of feeds a day down to eight. Let's say they can get a full feed in 20 minutes now, instead of 30, so that takes up less than three hours of their day. They might be able to stay awake for 30-45 minutes at a time during the day between naps. This is when you're starting to really see patterns with your baby's eating and sleeping routine. They may wake, eat for 20 minutes, spend 30 minutes awake with you, then fall asleep again. This is almost an hour of awake time.

Do you see how much time you gained when your baby pushed out their feeding schedule? Instead of spending six hours a day on feeds you're spending less than half that!

With more time between feeds this also gives your baby the opportunity for longer naps. If your baby feeds every hour and it takes 30 minutes to eat, the longest a nap will ever be is 30 minutes.

Once your baby can go four hours between feeds it's a game-changer. It's like your whole day frees up.

Below is a simple guide to how long a baby typically sleeps in a 24-hour period based on different ages.

- Newborns   16-20 hours/day   No nap predictability.
- 3-6 months   15-18 hours/day   3 naps
- 6-12 months   14-16 hours/day   2-3 naps

- 12-18 months   14-15 hours/day   1-2 naps

- 18-24 months   13-15 hours/day   1 nap

- 2-5 years   11-13 hours/day   0-1 nap

As you can see, the sleep needs of your baby decreases with age. They need to sleep less each day as the number of naps decreases. One simple thing to remember about naps, is keep the middle one (the lunchtime nap) the longest. A short morning nap, a long afternoon nap, and another short late afternoon nap will keep you on a pretty good schedule. Even if you don't have a set time for each nap, remember having a flexible routine is good for your baby. Short, long, short for naps - Morning, afternoon, late afternoon.

As you can see from the chart above, around 9-12 months, a baby may drop to two naps. The first one to go is the late afternoon nap. So, you have a short morning nap and a long afternoon nap. But how do you know they're ready to drop that third nap? They may not be tired at bedtime, or you may start to see too many nighttime wake ups.

Then, around 18 months, they may be ready to drop the morning nap. They may not be tired in the morning anymore. Or you may start to see really early wake ups, like 5 am.

Your child only needs so many hours of sleep in a 24-hour period. So, assuming they are sleeping well all night, as they get older, they need less sleep. If your one-year-old needs around 15 hours of sleep every day, they will likely sleep 12 hours at night, have a 30-minute morning nap, and the long afternoon nap will be around two hours. A two-year-old who needs 13 hours of sleep likely will sleep 12 hours at night with an hour afternoon nap. If your two-year-old doesn't need 13 hours, they may sleep 11 hours overnight with a one- to 1.5-hour nap. Listening and watching here is important to understand your particular child's sleep needs. If they get too much sleep overnight, they likely won't nap. You'll see them become very cranky in the evening and probably fall asleep at the dinner table. If they are sleeping too long during the day, they will be down to party at 10 p.m. and it will be hard to get them to bed at a reasonable hour.

If you're having trouble getting your child to sleep, hire a sleep consultant. You'll notice your child is sleep deprived if they are always tired, fall asleep at random times, are clumsy and get hurt often, can't concentrate, get headaches, have trouble at school, or can't regulate their moods. These are all signs that your child may not be getting enough rest.

Typically, by age four or five, most kids have kicked naps altogether. Sometimes a four-year-old may need a nap one day but not the next. This will likely mean they need an early bedtime that night. Young children still have sleep cues (usually extreme emotions), so watch that and get them to bed early if needed. When in doubt, early bedtime!

Sleep Environment

A dedicated sleep space is important. Many parents think, or have heard, that you have to let your baby fall asleep anywhere, so they get used to sleeping anywhere. This actually is not optimal for your baby's sleep. When a baby is sleeping in a living room and waking up every 30 minutes, they never get into a deep sleep state. Also, as they get older and start to produce their own sleep hormones (between six and nine weeks), they need daylight during wake time and darkness during sleep. Allowing them to sleep in open, bright, and noisy rooms does not actually give them better sleep.

Reminder here that the longer your baby sleeps for naps, the more time you have to do things that you need or want to do. If your baby only ever sleeps for 30 minutes at a time, you barely have time to shower and get dressed before you're at it again. Imagine all the things you can do during a two-hour nap!

So, what is an optimal sleep environment?

No matter where your baby sleeps, in a crib in the nursery or a bassinet in your room, the room should be dark. Minimize light from windows, night lights, monitors, and lamps. Use blinds, curtains, or blackout shades for naps and bedtime, especially in the summer months when it is light later. This applies to naps and bedtime. We don't just need darkness at night for sleep. When you put your baby or toddler down for a nap, make it dark in the room.

Our bodies need darkness to produce melatonin, the hormone that makes us feel sleepy. When the sun rises, our bodies warm and the light produces serotonin which makes us feel awake and energetic. That is a very simple way to explain an extremely complex biological process, but I just want you to understand that we, as humans, need both darkness and light for optimal sleep.

So, when the sun rises and warms us, we wake up. Most of us wake if we get too warm in the night. A dark, cool room, around 67 degrees, is ideal. Every house is different, so adjust as needed. An older, drafty home may feel too cold at 67 degrees. Some may feel warm, but most will be perfect between 66 and 68 degrees at night. This does not mean you have to keep your home set at that temperature all day. I would be freezing!

Air circulation is also important for optimal and safe sleep. If you have a ceiling fan in the nursery, keep it on low. If you have a tabletop fan, make sure it isn't blowing directly on the baby. Direct it toward the middle of the room just to keep air circulating. If you're worried about your baby being too hot or too cold, put them to bed then check on them after a half hour. Sometimes a baby's face, hands, or feet may feel cold, but check their core temperature. If their tummy or back feels warm, they are OK. If they feel hot and sweaty, you need to turn the heat down or remove a layer. It's not necessary to bundle your baby in multiple layers for sleep, nor is it safe. Remember, if we get too warm we wake up. We want to eliminate any reason for your baby waking early so a onesie and a sleep sack or swaddle is usually sufficient.

Sound is also important for optimal sleep. When a baby is in utero, it's noisy. They can hear your heart beating and your blood swooshing. Use a sound machine to recreate a constant, static noise in their sleep space. Turn it up fairly loud so that if a door slams, a dog barks, or the garbage truck rolls by outside, your baby won't hear it. Don't keep it right next to your baby. Place it on a dresser or table across the room. Find something with a rain, wave, or static sound that is soothing. No music or anything with birds chirping. The different tones and varying volumes can be distracting and wake a baby up.

Safe Sleep

Your baby should sleep on their back on a flat surface. Period. No blankets, stuffed animals, bumpers, or other loose objects in the sleeping area. No sleeping overnight in car seats or swings. A flat surface means a crib or bassinet with a hard, flat mattress and a fitted crib sheet. That's it.

Notice I said "no sleeping overnight" in car seats or swings. It will undoubtedly happen in a car seat on a car ride, but when you get home, you need to take your baby out of the car seat and transfer them to the crib or bassinet where it is safest.

Beware of inclined sleepers. There are several reasons you aren't supposed to use rockers or swings for sleep. They aren't considered safe and are constantly being recalled due to infant injury or death. You also don't want your baby to get used to only sleeping in a swing or you may have a really hard time getting them into the crib eventually.

Most parents will swaddle their newborns. Babies love this because in utero, they are snug and tight. A swaddle recreates that feeling of security. You may have to find a swaddle or position that your baby likes, but don't give up on it. You may have to swaddle your baby with arms up, arms down, one arm out. You figure out what your baby prefers. Typically, newborns prefer arms swaddled down, but as they get older they may have a different preference.

Swaddling also helps with the Moro Reflex, or startle reflex. This is when your baby suddenly jerks their limbs while sleeping and that wakes them up. For safe sleep, swaddling has to stop once your baby is rolling. We don't want your baby to be strapped with their arms into a swaddle and then roll to their tummy, trapped there. Once your baby can roll consistently, an arms-free swaddle is fine (both arms out), but if you're doing that, a swaddle is kind of useless. They can just wear a sleep sack or pajamas.

Sleep Cycles

Sleep cycles are another very complex topic but I'm going to break it down as simply as I can because it's important to understand what they are so you know what's happening in your little baby's brain and body. An adult sleep cycle is about 90 minutes. We cycle through REM and non-REM sleep several times until we wake up. At the end of a sleep cycle, we may wake up during the night. Most of the time you probably don't even remember. If you do, it may be when you adjusted your pillow or changed positions, then fell back asleep.

A baby's sleep cycle is only 45 minutes. Getting through a full sleep cycle is important for sleep otherwise your baby doesn't get through full REM and non-REM sleep. We need both, but it's especially important for this little human who is growing at a rapid pace. They need sleep[25] to grow, to build their immune systems, to regulate moods, to store memories, and for cognitive development. Without going on and on, I want you to understand that sleep is so very important for your growing baby. Getting through a full 45-minute sleep cycle is key, and as your baby gets older (remember when I said they will eventually be able to go four hours between feeds?) they will take a long afternoon nap. This nap should be two to three hours, which means they are going through a few sleep cycles. They cannot ever get a nap this long if they are hungry, that's why I talk about getting full feeds so much. They also may not ever get a nap this long if they are sleeping in a bright, noisy living room.

A baby who wakes up after 30 minutes consistently is, without a doubt, sleep deprived. A young baby who wakes up after 45 minutes consistently is making it through a full sleep cycle and will just need some assistance getting from one sleep cycle into the next when they are developmentally ready.

After a baby wakes from a 45-minute cycle, they may just need to be patted or rubbed while in the crib to fall back asleep. This is when you will hear them stir in the crib. They may cry for a bit, or moan and wiggle around. You will wait and watch. Oftentimes babies just need to fuss around for five minutes, then fall back asleep. If your baby fusses for a while and isn't able to fall back asleep, that's when you assist. Remember, we're talking about older babies here, let's say eight weeks and older in general. Not that you can't do this with younger babies, but as a general rule by two-months-old, most babies have a pretty predictable routine. When they wake from that sleep cycle, you know they don't need a feed because you just fed them before they went down for a nap. It's only been 45 minutes, they fussed around for 4 minutes and you notice they are going to start crying. Go in and assist without taking the baby out of the crib. I have a YouTube video on the Gold Coast Doulas channel called Shush Pat[26]. It's the best, and my favorite method for assisting small babies back to sleep. If your baby doesn't like shush pat, make up your own version. Hold their tummy and gently rock them back and forth until they settle. I used to run my finger lightly down my daughter's nose and across her forehead while I rocked her back and forth in the crib. At 10-years-old, she still loves it when I caress her forehead.

Assisting is your first step to teaching your baby to self-soothe. Why do you want to do this? Well, because then you aren't required to get them back to sleep every time by picking up, rocking, bouncing, feeding, or driving around in your car.

I've seen it all!

I had a client with an 18-month-old who needed to be driven around for well over an hour to fall asleep. Then imagine the parents' fear when the child finally fell asleep and now they had to get him out of the car seat and into the crib. They drove around for quite a while after just to make sure he was fully asleep. And they were exhausted, too. Yikes!

If you want to feed or rock your baby to sleep, do it! Just keep in mind that any habits you create now while your baby is small will likely carry through for several more months, if not years. You have to have the desire and the stamina to follow that through. There's nothing wrong with it as long as it's working for everyone. And by everyone, I mean you, your partner, and your baby.

Parents, I want to remind you here to be respectful and supportive of others' choices. Especially if you have a baby who sleeps well. Don't offer advice unless asked. There's nothing worse than a sleep-deprived parent enduring story after story of another parent's success. If they ask for advice, offer it. If they don't, ask how you can help but generally keep your opinion to yourself.

Sleep Tips

Listen Before You Intervene

I mentioned before that some babies make strange noises, especially at night. Baby noises during sleep are normal. There's no need to jump out of bed immediately. Remember how we learned to listen? Is your baby just waking from a sleep cycle, rustling around, and will fall back asleep on their own in a few minutes? Did they cry out briefly, fuss a bit, then settle back down? You'll never know if you rush over immediately. Give your baby the opportunity to put themselves back to sleep first. Wait and listen, then intervene when you know they need you.

Listen for intermittent noises. Did your baby cry for a brief period, then stop? Fuss for a bit, then yawn and go silent before fussing again? These are all normal noises a baby makes when waking from a sleep cycle and will often fall back to sleep on their own. If crying is persistent, intervene. If fussing is turning to crying, intervene. But if it's on and off, most babies just like to hear themselves chat for a while. Especially the light fussing and grunting sounds. These are the most common sleep noises. The toddler version of this will be singing or talking to themselves in bed while they hold on to their favorite stuffed animal.

If you know your baby eats every three hours and it's been two hours and 45 minutes, there's no need to wait and listen. It's a pretty sure bet that your baby is hungry so go in right away and feed him or her.

Consistency

Regardless of whether you consider yourself to be routine-oriented, most will find that having some consistency in their day is ideal, for them and their baby. Creating a consistent wake time, consistent bedtime, consistent naps, and consistent feed times is the simplest place to start. If you plan to feed on demand, you would just stick to a consistent wake time and bedtime. Nap times will be in between feeds but will not be consistent because you won't know when the next feed will be.

7 a.m. and 7 p.m. are very common wake and bedtimes. Anywhere between 6:30 and 7:30 is conducive to a child's natural circadian rhythm. One of the most common things I hear from sleep clients is that their baby's bedtime is 10 or 11 p.m. When I ask questions, I find out that the baby does in fact go to sleep around 7 p.m. but the parents just consider it a nap. When their baby wakes after 45 minutes, they get them up instead of helping them into another sleep cycle.

Early to bed

10 p.m. is far too late for a baby to be going to bed. Would you put a 5-year-old to bed that late? Probably not. Most 10-year-olds are going to bed around 8 or 9 pm still, so a newborn at 7 p.m. is not out of the question. This just gets hard for a family with two parents working outside the home. They may not get home until 6 p.m. and they will feel rushed to get quality time in with their baby before bed. In this instance, I ask clients what time they have to be up and out of the house. If it's not until later, like 9 a.m., I tell them that they can probably try an 8 p.m. bedtime and 8 a.m. wake time for their baby. But typically working households are up and out of the house early, which means baby has to be up early too. In that case, it means an early bedtime. These families have to focus on the quality time they get with their baby on the weekends, mornings, and the hour before bed.

Make sleep a priority

A well-rested baby is typically a healthy and happy baby who eats well and has a pleasant disposition throughout the day. This allows for more quality time during the day together. For working parents, I stress the importance of this quality time on the weekends. On the other hand, for babies that stay up late and don't nap well, they are typically tired and grumpy throughout the day. Sometimes they don't eat well and fight going down for naps. This makes it hard for parents to have quality time with their baby any day of the week.

Again, these are all very personal decisions and only you can make them. You know what's best for your family, but I want to put all the scenarios out there so you are informed and can make the best decision. My hope is that you can find or create a routine of your own that works for your family and your baby. Sometimes we get so caught up in what we need, what we want, or what our work schedules demand, that we don't consider what our baby needs.

Twins, Triplets, and Beyond

If you are having multiples, I want to remind you that a routine is really important. You want your babies to be sleeping at the same time or you'll never get a break. Remember, it's really important to have help in your home at first with multiples. With twins or triplets, having a set of hands for each baby is helpful. You'll want to feed them all at the same time and get them down for naps at the same time. Staggered feeds and naps will be never-ending for you.

Keep in mind that with twins and triplets, you will try to get them on a consistent schedule but realize that they are different humans with different personalities, temperaments, and sleep needs. With time you may find that one baby is an early riser, and the other takes shorter naps. A sleep consultant can be a real asset here.

Day and Night

We talked a bit about sleep cycles, but let's talk a little more about the importance of daylight and darkness. During daylight hours, while your baby is awake, try to keep them active. Even if they're only awake for 10 minutes, sit by a window, set them on a play mat, or get outside. Active play during wake times is so important especially as they get older.

Another tip about daylight is try to feed in a bright room. Unless it's nighttime, we don't want your baby eating in the dark or they will likely fall asleep. Our goal with feeds is to get a full feed. If it's dark, you're signaling to your baby's brain that it is sleep time. But if you feed in a well-lit room, the sunlight will hopefully keep your baby awake longer, which in turn leads to a longer feed, which leads to a full belly, which leads to longer sleep. Phew!

After a full feed, try to keep your baby awake for a bit in the light. Remember at first your newborn will probably fall asleep at the breast or bottle. Then they might be able to stay awake for five minutes, then 15, then 45, and so on. We want feeds to happen in a well-lit room, then active play time in daylight, then sleep in a dark room. The sooner you can separate the act of feeding from sleeping, the better for sleep hygiene. Unless, of course, you want to feed your baby to sleep (sometimes for a very long time!). This becomes the main part of the routine which will have to be repeated throughout the night in order to get your baby to fall asleep again. This decision will depend on your parenting style, if you work, where your baby sleeps, and how much sleep you want to get at night. If you don't want to feed your baby to sleep, separating those two activities will be key.

When your baby is in active playtime, it's important to learn your baby's sleep cues here. You may notice they start to yawn, rub their eyes, cry, whine, chatter to themselves, or get really excited (usually before a crash). Notice and understand these cues because it's your baby communicating with you. They are telling you they are starting to get tired, and you have a small window of time. Get them into their sleep space, dim the lights, and have a little bit of wind down time. You can even get them into pjs if you want. When the nap is over, open the shades and let the sun in. This will help wake your baby up naturally.

So put this all together and what does it look like? After a full feed in daylight, your baby will get tired during active playtime, then you put them to bed. Your baby just got a full feed, active time in daylight which wore them out, and now they are ready for bed. And because you are so good at watching their cues, you knew they were getting tired and put them into the crib right away. Good job!

Just as we want active playtime in daylight, we want darkness for all sleep times. Our brains produce serotonin in the light, and darkness turns serotonin to melatonin to make us feel sleepy. That means even for naps during the day, we want your baby to sleep in a dark room. Pull the curtains, turn the sound machine on, cuddle and sing a song, then get your baby into the crib while they're drowsy. Rock them back and forth in the crib, rub their belly, and help guide them to sleep in the crib. This is your ideal situation. In reality, most of you will be rocking, bouncing, or feeding your baby to sleep. Remember if you can separate feeds from sleep, and get your baby used to falling asleep safely on their back in the crib without you doing much, they are essentially falling asleep in the crib on their own. This means, most of the time when they wake in the night from a sleep cycle, they will be able to put themselves back to sleep without needing you, unless it's time to eat. And if they do need you, you just have to rock them back and forth in the crib for a bit, which is a lot less time consuming than picking up, rocking, and feeding back to sleep.

Don't keep a night light by the crib or have noisy or light up mobiles nearby. If you need a light to see in the night to feed or change a diaper, consider a light on a dimmer switch, or a night light you turn on low only when needed.

Listen and Learn

Do you have a dog? Have you noticed your dog also communicates with you? They have different barks and different things they do to let you know what they need or want. My dog has very distinct barks. If I let him out in the backyard, I know his bark when he's cornered a squirrel up a tree. I know his bark when the neighbor dogs are out and on the other side of the fence. I know his bark when he is on the leash, caught on a bush, and needs help. I also know his bark when he's ready to come back inside. To a non-dog owner, a bark may just sound like a bark. But we know that's not true.

This is the same for your baby. As your baby grows, their cries and cues will change. All cries are not the same nor do they mean the same thing.

Bedtime Routines

This is one of the most important and fun parts of a sleep schedule! If you create a consistent routine from the beginning, you'll be set for years to come. We typically think about bedtime routines as being important for older children, but it's great for you to create a routine for your baby right away.

A typical routine goes much like this: feed, change diaper, put on pjs, read a book, dim the lights, sing a song, turn on the sound machine, and put baby into the crib or bassinet. Notice how feeding is separate from sleeping. I'll say it again, the sooner you can make those two activities separate, the better. If you end up having to nurse to get your baby to fall asleep, that means every time your baby wakes up from a sleep cycle in the night, you may have to nurse them back to sleep. Remember, a sleep cycle is 45 minutes so that doesn't allow you much time to sleep in between feeds. Once again, if you feed to sleep and it works for you then by all means continue! It's only a problem if you think it is!

For many families this doesn't work and is often the reason they call me for help. It's such an easy bind to get yourself in because in the beginning your baby almost always falls asleep at the breast or bottle. If you don't plan to do this but it happens anyway, you haven't failed or done anything wrong. Try some of the tips I mentioned and if you can't do it alone, find a sleep consultant to guide you through it gently.

As your baby gets more efficient at feeding and you notice a feeding routine forming, try to start shifting more feeds during the day and fewer at night. Your baby only needs so many calories in one day. Start to focus on having less calorie intake at night. This is easier to understand for bottle fed babies. Let's say a bottle-fed baby eats 28 ounces a day and feeds every three hours. That's eight feeds a day with 3.5 ounces per feed. If you can shift daytime feeds to four ounces you can start to slowly eliminate night feeds. Here's what I mean:

- 7 a.m.   4-ounce feed
- 10 a.m.   4-ounce feed
- 1 p.m.   4-ounce feed
- 4 p.m.   4-ounce feed
- 7 p.m.   4-ounce feed

Your baby has now taken 20 ounces during the day, and you know it need 28. That leaves only eight ounces overnight. In a perfect world, your baby would wake only twice in the night for two four-ounce feeds. That's seven feeds total at four ounces instead of eight at 3.5 ounces. You've just eliminated one night feed!

You may find your baby can't take 4 ounces yet. Don't force it or rush it. Try again in a week or two. Or you may find that in the morning they will take four, 3.5 the rest of the day, and four ounces again before bed. Every little bit counts. Your baby still gets the same calories in a 24-hour period, they're just getting more during the day and less at night. You will have to experiment here and figure out when your baby is ready for this. Bigger feeds during the day means they need less at night, which allows for longer stretches of night sleep. Why? Because they aren't waking up hungry!

When your baby wakes from a sleep cycle during a nap or at night and you know they don't need a feed, try listening and waiting. If they don't fall back to sleep on their own, try patting them, rocking them back and forth in the crib, rubbing their belly, or shushing them in the crib. Trying all these first will allow them the opportunity to fall back to sleep on their own without you having to rock, feed, or bounce them back to sleep. Soon you'll be on your way to a full night's sleep!

Sleep myths

I love dispelling weird myths and misconceptions we've heard about sleep. So many times, I'll hear someone repeat something their mother or grandmother told them about sleep and it's usually nonsense.

Sleep Myth #1 - Don't wake a sleeping baby

False. Newborns love to sleep and may decide they want to sleep through a feed. You will want to wake your newborn to feed if it's been over three hours (we talked about this, remember?). They need to eat. Their growing bodies need the nutrients. Also, as naps become more regular, an older baby that wants to take a three-hour nap in the morning should be woken up. That's far too long for a morning nap. You want to focus on the afternoon nap being the longest as they get older. If you let your baby sleep three hours in the morning, you'll start to see them to wake up for the day very early... like 4 a.m. Ouch.

Check the cheat sheet below for age-appropriate wake times. You don't want your baby sleeping too much during the day. They won't be tired at bedtime and will also wake frequently in the night. But you also don't want to try to keep them awake too long or they will become overly tired and fight sleep. It's a delicate balance, and a sleep consultant can be beneficial here as well. She can figure out the best nap schedule for your baby based on age.

How long should my baby stay awake between naps?

- 0-3 weeks: 5-30 minutes awake. Feeding frequently.
- 3-6 weeks: 40-75 minutes awake. Feeding frequently and more predictably.
- 7-11 weeks: 90 minutes awake. Feeding every 2-3 hours.
- 3 months: 1 hour 45 min awake. 4-5 hrs daily naps, 3 naps/day. Eating every 3-3.5 hrs.
- 4 months: 2 hours awake. 4 hrs daily naps, 3 naps, feeding every 4 hours.

- 5 months: 2 hrs 15 min awake. 3.5 hrs daily naps, 3 naps.
- 6 months: 2.5 hours awake, 3 hrs daily sleep with 3 naps. Starting solids.

This chart is important to show us why we may want to wake a sleeping baby. If your baby sleeps too long, they probably won't be tired at bedtime.

Here's a scenario of a sleep schedule going awry:

Baby wakes at 7 a.m. and feeds. This baby is four-months-old and can stay awake for about two hours before needing to sleep again. That means the first nap should be around 9 a.m. Unfortunately, you were busy doing something else, missed baby's sleep cues, and tried to put baby down for a nap at 9:45. Your baby is now overly tired and fights sleep. You finally get baby down to sleep at 10:30 but they wake up again at 11 because it's time to eat. This means the next nap should be around 1 p.m. but they are overly tired now and can't make it. They show sleep signs at noon, so you put them down again. This time they sleep for one hour and are awake at 2 p.m. This puts the next nap around 4. They make it until 4 p.m. and fall asleep right away. You notice it's 6 p.m. and your baby is still sleeping so you figure "they need it" and let them keep sleeping. They wake at 6:30 hungry so you feed them. Now it's only 30 minutes until their bedtime but they just woke up from a nap! Without a doubt, this baby is going to have very disrupted overnight sleep with a lot of wake ups and an early wake time, probably around 5 or 6 a.m.

Ideally this four-month-old would have a short nap in the morning at 9 a.m, a nice long 2.5-hour nap in the afternoon, and another short nap in the late afternoon. If any of those naps goes too long and you don't wake them, it disrupts the whole day, and you'll see the nighttime go awry as well.

It's OK to wake a sleeping baby!

Sleep Myth #2 - I have to let my baby cry it out

False! No! If your baby is hungry or ill, no amount of crying will help them sleep. This just causes unnecessary distress for you and them.

But… crying is normal. It's the only way your baby can communicate. Remember, you learned they do communicate. Once you can distinguish what their cries mean, you will be able to respond accordingly. We also talked before about listening. This builds trust between you and your baby. If they cry because they are hungry, you give them food. If they cry because they are hurt, you pick them up and help them. If they are tired, you put them to bed. Most babies have a tired cry. They fuss and cry for a bit, wiggle around in the crib, and if left to figure it out on their own for a short while, will go back to sleep. Listen and figure out what your baby is telling you before you intervene. This absolutely does not mean you leave your baby to cry it out.

Crying it out means you leave your baby to cry until they fall asleep. This is unnecessary and teaches them nothing (and is excruciating for parents). Small bouts of crying or fussing is not letting them cry it out because you are there listening, ready to intervene when necessary. You are not shutting the door and walking away for the night.

A small amount of crying is normal. And once you've learned the skill of listening, you'll likely notice your baby cries for a bit, and can fuss themselves back to sleep without your help. In the early days, they will need your assistance (patting in the crib, shushing, and if necessary, picking up).

If anyone ever suggests that you need to just leave your baby or child in the crib, walk away, and let them cry it out, seek advice from someone else.

Sleep Myth #3 - Keep them up during the day so they sleep at night

False. Adult sleep rules do not apply to babies. Keeping them up all day will create over tiredness which actually disrupts nighttime sleep even more. Remember what you just learned about age-appropriate awake windows? If you notice tired signs, that means your baby is tired, so put them to bed.

Tired signs could include obvious ones like yawning or eye rubbing. But for some babies, especially as they get older and more vocal, becoming very loud, chatty, or excitedly banging toys can be a tired sign. Oftentimes parents will think they are very awake when they are just about to crash. It's important to notice these signs right away and get them to bed before they become overly tired and fight sleep.

Babies, and older children, need more sleep than most parents expect. We are raising a generation of sleep-deprived children.

Parents' Sleep

Most parents after having a baby wonder if they will ever sleep again. When families call me for help it's been several months, and sometimes years, of very little sleep. Most parents can't function this way. The sleep deprivation wears on you physically, mentally, and relationships suffer. I've seen marriages on the brink of divorce because children are sleeping in the parent's bed, while one parent has been sleeping in the spare bedroom or on a mattress on the floor. I've seen sleep-deprived mothers wonder if they will ever get their lives back. They haven't seen friends, have had no time alone, and have done nothing for themselves in so long. I've seen mothers and partners struggle at work because their sleep deprivation is so intense.

I want to make sure you know that, yes, you will sleep. Some of you will struggle more than others. Some of you may have a hard time asking for help. No matter what your sleep journey looks like, always know that you're doing the best you can. You've done nothing "the wrong way" and you haven't ruined your children. Everyone will be good. Ask for help when you need it. And if someone offers help, don't be too proud to take it.

For those of you having a baby with a toddler at home, the best thing to do is get your toddler on a good schedule now! If you have time and patience, start working on it while you're pregnant. Set up a good bedtime routine, stay consistent, and if you can't figure it out, seek professional help from a sleep consultant.

Quick Tips for Toddler Sleep

Typically, a toddler is down to one nap a day in the afternoon. Depending on the sleep needs of your particular child this nap may be one to two hours. This will also depend on how much overnight sleep they get. Apply what you now know about a consistent routine to your toddler's schedule. Set a consistent wake time and a consistent bedtime. Also keep a consistent nap time in the afternoon.

For instance, a toddler's nap is typically between one and three p.m. Your toddler may only sleep an hour, but two is typical. Don't let the nap go over three hours unless they are sick.

Why?

What did we learn about sleeping too long for a nap? Your toddler won't be tired for bedtime if you let them sleep four hours in the afternoon.

Most kids need about 12 to 14 hours of sleep per day. You will have to watch your child to know how much they need. If your toddler sleeps 12 hours at night from 7 p.m. to 7 a.m., and no matter how hard you try you cannot get them to take a two-hour nap, they probably need 13 hours of sleep in a day. Twelve hours overnight and one hour for a nap. If you really need that two-hour stretch, you could try to cut down overnight sleep by an hour and add it to the nap. For instance, 7:30 p.m. to 6:30 a.m. overnight with a two-hour nap at 1 p.m.

Every child is different, so you have to be patient while trying out a new schedule.

Give it a few days and see how it works for your child. Trying something once doesn't work. Some kids take two days to fall into a new routine, while some of our more feisty kids may take a week. You know your child; give them the time they need. Be gentle but be consistent.

Don't go it alone; hire a sleep consultant if you find you're struggling with sleep. Find one that is reputable. That means no cry-it-out consultants. They should have references or testimonials from other parents.

They know several different methods and will choose the best one for your family. If they only know and use one method, find someone else.

There is no one-size-fits-all sleep solution. That's why you can't just read one book or take an online course and expect perfect results. You might get lucky and that one method you learned about is the best one for your baby or toddler, but more than likely you'll need to use a combination of several different methods based on how your child responds, and their evolving temperament.

The sleep consultant should also take your parenting style into consideration. Sleep training gets a bad rap! If only parents knew that they could hire sleep help and it wouldn't be scary, they would do it in a heartbeat. So many of my clients say they wished they hadn't waited so long. They were scared because of all the misconceptions (for example Cry It Out or super rigid schedules) so they kept trying things themselves that obviously didn't work, until they finally gave up and called for help. It breaks my heart to hear the tears over the phone. I can hear the sleep deprivation in their voices and how it's affecting them.

Sleep is critical to your mental wellness as a new parent. Sleep helps increase breastmilk production and boosts your immunity. This is mostly because of the stress caused by sleep deprivation.[27] Stress can wreak havoc on our bodies. For your baby[28], sleep is critical for brain development, emotional regulation, and physical growth. It also helps build their immune system.

Remind yourself that sleep is one of the most important elements of your wellbeing and your baby's development. It's free, there are no negative side effects, and it's proven to do wonders. Make it a priority!

SLEEP STORIES

🗩 Sleep Stories by Alyssa

"Even before I became a sleep consultant, I was obsessed with sleep, and still am. I need my sleep or I transform into a werewolf. Not really, but I feel like one. Because I love my sleep so much, I knew I needed to get my daughter into a good sleep routine, and I started right away. She and I were both getting great sleep early on, so we were able to really enjoy our awake time together. A well-rested mother is happier and healthier, and same with a well-rested baby. My daughter would wake up smiling and I was always happy to greet her! This created more quality time when we were together, and I cherished every moment.

"Bed-sharing with my baby did not equal attachment and bonding for me; my daughter slept in her crib and I in my bed. In order for me to be capable of bonding, I needed rest. I was a much better mother because I knew my limits, starting with healthy sleep habits early, and forming healthy bonds and attachments with my daughter while she was awake, not asleep."

🗩 Sleep Stories from Dominique Tol, Gold Coast sleep client

"Before we reached out to Alyssa for a sleep consultation, it was getting to a point where our seven-month-old daughter wasn't taking naps, and if she was taking naps, it was for 15 minutes at a time. She was fussy all day. We were having to rock her to sleep for every single nap and bedtime. It took 20 minutes to get her to take a 15-minute nap!

"It was getting to a point where she didn't seem like she was getting good sleep, and we were getting so frustrated. I read a lot about crying-it-out and how it increases cortisol levels in babies so they're stressed out. I was like, well, I don't want to do that! I don't want to set her up for not wanting to reach out to us for comfort, but it also seemed like she was not happy during the day. She was fussy and irritable all the time because she wasn't sleeping well. I was so worried about her crying at night, but she was crying all day anyway. So, I was like, OK, there's got to be some other ways to do this.

"We saw results the first night of sleep training. Instead of rocking her for 20 minutes, we did her bedtime routine, which was a new thing that we incorporated. Instead of nursing her to sleep, I was nursing her and then we would change into pajamas, wash her face, read her a book, and then put her to bed. That very first night, we laid her down, and she started crying. We waited three minutes, and then went in for 30 seconds to soothe her while lying in her crib without taking her out. I think it was two rounds of that. So, she cried for three minutes; I went in; she cried for another three minutes; I went in; and then it was quiet in her room.

"I looked over at my husband, and I was like, this can't be real! It was amazing. She went to sleep, and I think that first night, she slept for about six hours, and then she got up to nurse, and then she went back to sleep fine.

"Letting her cry for a few minutes in her crib ended up being way less than she cried during the day. That little bit of crying was what she needed to learn to soothe herself to sleep. We felt good about it. It wasn't like we felt like we were neglecting her by letting her cry in her crib. She put herself to sleep, and now she's getting a good chunk of sleep. We have a baby that sleeps well and is so much happier during the day!"

📋 Sleep Consultant Wisdom from Alyssa

Get yourself on a consistent sleep schedule now while pregnant. If sleep is hard to come by, carry out the routine with rest. Try to get at least eight hours of sleep a night and once baby arrives, track your sleep in a journal or in an app on your phone. That means if you've only had three hours of sleep in a night, you will have to cancel visits from friends and reschedule lunch dates. Why? So, you can take a nap! Don't overbook yourself. Focus on your health, healing, and bonding with your baby. All of this is easier when you've had enough sleep.

CHAPTER 11

Your Mental Health

We decided to reach out to Cristina Stauffer, LMSW, for expert advice in this chapter. Cristina was in Kristin's Sacred Pregnancy class and later taught infant massage for Gold Coast Doulas. She is a private practice psychotherapist who specializes in supporting clients experiencing infertility, miscarriage and infant loss, pregnancy complications, perinatal mood and anxiety disorders and the adjustment to parenthood in general.

Observations from Cristina Stauffer...

Welcome to the wonderful, and sometimes terrifying, world of parenthood.

Not feeling like yourself?

That is to be expected. Becoming a parent is one of the biggest emotional transitions you are likely to make. But when does your mood look or feel like something that might need more attention? Let's talk for a bit about the emotional adjustment to motherhood, postpartum depression, and everything that goes along with maternal mental health.

As an outpatient psychotherapist who specializes in supporting families through the transition to parenthood, I get a lot of questions about postpartum depression and what is "normal". Here some of the most common questions I hear:

"I can't stop crying! I don't even feel sad and there is nothing wrong, but I am just so emotional. What is happening to me?"

If these symptoms are occurring within the first two weeks after giving birth, they are most likely the "baby blues". Almost all women will experience some tearfulness and emotional dysregulation as their bodies and hormones adjust from the event of giving birth. If these feelings last longer than two weeks after birth, they might indicate something more. Reach out to your medical provider or a trained therapist or counselor for further assessment.

"This can't be postpartum depression, can it? But I love my baby!"

There is a common misconception that having postpartum depression means that you do not feel connected to your baby. Although that can be a symptom of postpartum depression, it is not usually the case. Most of the women who I have worked with love and want their baby very much but just do not feel like themselves or like they are being the kind of mother they expected themselves to be.

"I have always had some depression and/or anxiety. How do I know if this is just my usual depression or postpartum depression?"

The true answer to this question is that it doesn't matter if you have a history of depression or anxiety or if this is your first experience with it. Treatment recommendations are the same either way. Past episodes of depression/anxiety or not, your coping skills and ability to use them change when you have a baby. No longer able to relax in the bath or concentrate on a good book? You are not alone. In some cases women even find that the medications they have used effectively do not work as well after they have had a baby. What is important is to seek treatment as soon as possible and to focus on what you need to feel better this time.

"I don't feel sad or depressed, but I am so worried and overwhelmed! I just can't relax or turn my brain off. What is going on?"

Anxiety is most likely to blame for these feelings. One of the most powerful things I have learned in my work with pregnant and postpartum women is that anxiety is far more common than depression. Women report feeling like they cannot let their guard down or allow themselves to relax. Feeling completely overwhelmed or like one is paralyzed to make a decision are also common experiences for women experiencing postpartum anxiety.

"This is not what I expected. I feel so sad and like I have made a terrible mistake. I don't even feel like this baby is mine. I am just the babysitter. What is wrong with me?"

Sometimes the adjustment to motherhood is not at all what we expect. Parents often are unprepared for the sense of loss they can experience, loss of self, loss of freedom, loss of spontaneity, loss of coping skills and outlets from their pre-child lifestyle. It is OK to not love every minute of motherhood. It is OK to love your baby and question your decision to become a parent at the same time. If postpartum depression is to blame for these feelings, you will get better with time and treatment. You have not missed your "window" of time to bond with your baby. You will get there. Be gentle with yourself and accept the support that you need.

"I am just so irritated! My partner is driving me crazy. No one can do anything right. I have such a short fuse that I could just punch someone. Why doesn't anyone understand me?"

Irritability is often a symptom of depression that is overlooked. Depression in the postpartum period tends to be a more irritated, agitated depression and less sad and withdrawn. Some women report even feeling rageful. Yes, postpartum rage is a real thing. Instead of identifying anger and irritability as a symptom, women often personalize it. "Why am I acting like this? Why am I so mean? I must be a terrible person." We need to shift the narrative to help women see irritability, anger, or rage as treatable symptoms, not a character flaw.

"I keep having these awful thoughts and/or images of something terrible happening to my baby! Who thinks these things? Am I some kind of a monster?"

Intrusive or obsessive thoughts can be a common experience for new parents. Almost all new parents report having unwanted thoughts of harm coming to their baby. What is most important to monitor is how much distress these thoughts are causing you. If you are able to dismiss them quickly by thinking something like "that was a weird thing to think about" or "that is not likely to ever happen", you are coping well with them. If you find yourself getting stuck thinking and worrying about these thoughts or changing your behavior to avoid things that might cause you to have an intrusive thought, you could be experiencing symptoms of postpartum obsessive-compulsive disorder.

Perinatal Mood and Anxiety Disorders (PMAD)

I know Alyssa touched on these briefly, but I will touch on them a little more. PMAD is an umbrella term for the various ways mental health symptoms can present themselves during pregnancy and the postpartum period. Postpartum depression is only one of the possible diagnoses on the continuum. Other diagnoses can include postpartum anxiety, postpartum obsessive-compulsive disorder, postpartum bipolar disorder, and postpartum psychosis.

Research has shown that 15-20 percent of women and 10 percent of men will experience symptoms in the perinatal period. Partners may not have the hormonal shifts that the birthing person experiences but their adjustment to parenthood can include loss of coping skills, grief over the loss of their old lifestyle, sleep deprivation, depression and anxiety.

PMAD can occur during pregnancy or days or months after childbirth. It is not uncommon to see women still struggling with symptoms into the second year of their child's life if their PMAD has gone untreated. Seeking treatment and support as soon as possible is best and can decrease the length of suffering.

PMAD Risk Factors

- Lack of social support; single parenting
- Personal or family history of mental illness
- Personal or family history of PMAD
- Marital or relationship conflict

- Poverty
- Stressful life events — loss of a loved one or a job, moving, divorce…
- Difficult or complicated pregnancy
- Traumatic labor and delivery experience
- Complications with the baby — NICU stay, medical concerns, etc
- Previous miscarriage or pregnancy loss
- History of infertility
- Poor sleep patterns or sleep deprivation
- Poor or inadequate nutrition
- Depression or anxiety during pregnancy

A note about women who have experienced pregnancy loss or infertility: These mamas often feel guilty if they do not love every minute of motherhood after working so hard to get pregnant or carry a pregnancy to term. They can feel tremendous guilt and shame if they experience any negative feelings about their motherhood experience. The truth is that you can love your baby/parenthood AND not enjoy every task, stage, or emotion. Parenting is hard no matter how much you want to be a parent.

Sometimes none of these risk factors are present and PMAD still occurs. Remember that PMAD does not discriminate and can happen to anyone and during or after any pregnancy. You are not to blame and with treatment you will get well.

Signs and Symptoms of PMAD

Depression

- Sadness and crying
- Irritability, having a short fuse
- Anger or rage
- Feeling overwhelmed
- Appetite and sleep changes

- Lack of feelings for the baby
- Unable to care for self or family
- Guilt and shame
- Feelings of hopelessness/helplessness
- Loss of interest and pleasure in things that usually bring you joy
- Suicidal thoughts

Anxiety

- Excessive worry
- Agitation
- Hypervigilance
- Sleep disturbance
- Poor appetite
- Racing thoughts
- Excessive concern about the health of baby or self

Postpartum Bipolar Disorder

Characterized by mood swings between:

- Depressive symptoms (as listed above)
- Mania (excessive energy, need for little sleep, pressured speech or fast talking, impulsivity, agitation, sometimes delusions/hallucinations)

The average age of onset for bipolar disorder is in the early 20s, which happens to coincide with peak reproductive years. Mood swings can be severe with intense episodes of mania (Bipolar I disorder) or more mild as characterized by hypomania (Bipolar II).

Postpartum Obsessive-Compulsive Disorder

- Obsessive thoughts or images often about harm coming to the baby
- Compulsive behavior or rituals - cleaning, checking, washing

Obsessive thoughts can also be called intrusive thoughts or scary thoughts. They are symptoms of anxiety and can be very distressing to those who experience them. Postpartum women often describe intrusive thoughts as being quite detailed and graphic or like they are seeing a quick clip of a movie in their mind. These thoughts can present as a "what-if" type of worry or a visual image of something terrible happening. Sometimes parents even see or think about themselves doing something terrible to the baby.

Intrusive thoughts are experienced as ego dystonic meaning that they are disturbing or distressing to the person experiencing them. Many mothers with postpartum OCD believe they have postpartum psychosis and are afraid to seek help. If you are upset by the thoughts you are having and recognize that they are not typical for you, you are most likely experiencing obsessive or intrusive thoughts and not postpartum psychosis.

A good rule is to remember to think about the level of distress the thoughts are causing you and not the fact that you are having them. A diagnosis of anxiety or OCD is based on how badly the obsessive (intrusive) thoughts are disrupting your daily life rather than on just experiencing the symptom itself.

Postpartum Psychosis (PPP)

Postpartum psychosis is very rare. Less than two out of every 1,000 postpartum women will develop postpartum psychosis. However, when it does occur it is a psychiatric emergency.

This condition has a rapid onset, usually within the first three weeks after delivery. It is characterized by a break with reality, sometimes drastic and sometimes subtle. Women may develop a religious preoccupation believing that they are being commanded to do things by a higher power, believe that they are receiving messages in other ways, or have intense or bizarre episodes of paranoia.

The media often does us a disservice by sensationalizing cases of postpartum psychosis. The reality is that of the small number of women who develop postpartum psychosis, only a very small percentage of them go on to commit infanticide or die by suicide. People often confuse the symptoms of postpartum psychosis with postpartum depression and are afraid to seek treatment because they think they are going "crazy" or will have their baby taken away from them.

The most important thing to remember about postpartum psychosis is that it is an emergency. If you suspect PPP, do not leave the mother unattended. Take her directly to the nearest emergency department or psychiatric crisis center for assessment.

Treatment and Recovery

Good news, mama! There are several ways to treat perinatal mood and anxiety disorders. You will recover. You will feel like yourself again in time, with the right support and care. There are several components to recovering from PMAD—therapy, medication, support, and self-care. You do not need to utilize all four things to get well, but know that using a combination of them may get you on the road to recovery faster.

- Improved self-care practices including utilizing support system more fully
- Support groups—peer lead or professional lead, online or in person
- Medication from primary care physician, OB/GYN, or psychiatrist
- Outpatient therapy with a therapist specially training in PMAD
- Partial or Inpatient Psychiatric Hospitalization for more extreme cases

I have listed multiple resources labeled "mental health" with websites and phone numbers in the **Trusted Resources** section at the end of this book.

PPD STORIES

🗩 PPD Story from Bri Luginbill, former Gold Coast photographer

"During pregnancy I struggled physically. I had a lot of sciatic nerve pain so in my third trimester I had weekly appointments with my DO just to get adjusted. My mental health was still OK at this time.

"As soon as I had my baby, it was a very stressful time. I had a lot of blood loss, and I almost hemorrhaged during delivery, so I think when I had my baby, I was just exhausted. I remember them putting him on me and thinking hey, there's a baby there, but not really feeling that instant love because I was just so tired. So, from that first interaction, although I was told I was supposed to feel instant love, instant excitement, I was just too worn out.

"When I went to the bathroom the first time, another blood clot passed. I almost passed out, and I remember telling the nurse, 'I can't hear anything, but I know you're there. I'm starting to lose my vision. I'm just letting you know.'

"On top of that, I have a family history of anxiety and depression, which I feel like is not a fair combination to have! You get anxious, and then your thoughts race, and then you feel bad about yourself, and then it's just like a cycle. Over time, I've learned some coping strategies to manage this. I am able to let people know that I'm feeling sad, anxious, or depressed.

"When I went home, I was anxious at night because I was worried about my baby and just wanted to make sure he was OK. Then I was depressed during the day because that anxiety wore me out. I talked to my doctor, and I did start taking medicine as soon as I could after getting out of the hospital because I had taken Zoloft before. I was doing all the things I knew of to try to deal with my feelings, but I wasn't being very compassionate to myself.

"My word of advice and encouragement to people is if you are feeling those feelings, as long as you're voicing them, getting help and asking for support, don't beat yourself up. You're already doing so much. You've entered into this whole new world with a tiny new person, and you deserve to be understanding to yourself, while trying to understand what's happening.

"The medicine seemed like it helped a little bit, but it was still like learning a new system, learning a new normal, learning what this means, and it really does take a village. I think what I've learned with having my baby is to let go of control more. I'll always be a planner, it's who I am, but I'm trying to let go of control more. I'm also working on having more self-compassion. Just being compassionate towards myself makes things a little bit less extreme and makes me less anxious."

📋 Doula Wisdom from Kristin

Don't be afraid to talk about how you are feeling with a medical professional, therapist, or your partner. There are many free in-person and virtual support groups as well. You don't have to do this alone. It isn't a sign of weakness to ask for help.

📋 Doula Wisdom from Alyssa

Remember that some initial feelings of sadness are normal. Feeling overwhelmed is normal. Don't automatically assume something is wrong or you're not good at being a mom. Have someone who knows you well ask how you're doing frequently and be honest with your answers. If these feelings don't go away or escalate to higher levels of sadness, fatigue, depression, or rage, ask for help! Tell someone. Talk to a friend or call your doctor's office. There's no award for doing this alone.

CHAPTER 12

You've Got This!

Wow! After all that, we just want you to know that this is your unique journey. You need to do what's best for you, your baby, your partner, and your growing family. Trust your instincts. Ask questions. Believe in yourself and know that you're going to be awesome at this parenting gig. Especially if you set yourself up for success with the right support people. We hope we've made it very clear why a team of support people matters. You do not have to do this alone! No matter who you are or where you live, how you choose to birth, or if this is your first or fifth, you have options. You have choices. Knowledge is power.

We are so happy you took this journey with us. If you ever want more info about support, services, or classes, please reach out. We'd love to have you join us in our "Becoming a Mother" course and answer your questions in person.

> *"Asking for help isn't giving up.*
> *It's refusing to give up."*
>
> — Charlie Mackesy, author of
> *The Boy, the Mole, the Fox, and the Horse*

Appendix - Trusted Resources

Apps

Baby Tracker
Count the Kicks
Wolomi
Expectful
WebMD Pregnancy
The Bump
ProDaddy (For Partners)
DLM App (Dysfunctional Labor Maneuvers)

Podcasts

Ask The Doulas
Informed Pregnancy Podcast
Plus Pregnancy
The Birth Hour
The Be Her Village Podcast
Happy Hour with Bundle Birth Nurses
Evidence Based Birth
Yoga Birth Babies
Birth Stories in Color
Dem Black Mamas Podcast
Respectful Parenting
The Motherly Podcast
The Birth Geeks' Podcast
Adventure Nannies On Air
NATAL

Registries

Poppylist www.poppylist.com
Babylist www.babylist.com

Amazon www.amazon.com
Target www.target.com
My Registry www.MyRegistry.com
Be Her Village www.behervillage.com

Sources for Finding A Doula and other Birth and Baby Experts

DoulaMatch www.doulamatch.net
National Black Doulas Association www.blackdoulas.org
Meela www.hellomeela.com
TotSquad www.totsquad.com, Find sleep consultants, lactation, car seat safety and more.
Bornbir www.bornbir.com
Okkanti www.okkanti.com
VBAC Doulas VBAC Academy www.vbacacademy.com

Nanny and NCS Agencies

Adventure Nannies www.adventurenannies.com
Educated Nannies www.educatednannies.com
Newborn Care Solutions www.newborncaresolutions.com

Doula Training Organizations (Some of our favorites)

ProDoula www.prodoula.com
CAPPA www.cappa.net
Bebo Mia www.bebomia.com
DONA www.dona.org
ICEA www.icea.org
National Black Doula Association www.blackdoulas.org
DTI www.wearedti.com

Plus Size Pregnancy Support

Plus Size Birth www.plussizebirth.com
Fat and Pregnant www.fatandpregnant.com

Multiples and NICU Support

FLRRISH www.flrrish.com, Navigating the NICU
Mothers of Multiples Society www.mothersofmultiples.com
Multiples of America www.multiplesofamerica.org

Surrogacy

Bright Futures Family www.brightfuturesfamilies.com
Worldwide Surrogacy www.worldwidesurrogacy.org/resources
Surrogacy Simplified www.surrogacysimplified.com

Newborn Care Specialist Training Orgs

Newborn Care Solutions www.newborncaresolutions.com
The Newborn Care Training Academy www.newborncaretraining.com

Pregnancy and Birth Decks/Cards

Mama Natural Pregnancy Affirmation Cards by Genevieve Howland.
The Fair Play Deck: A Couple's Conversation Deck for
    Prioritizing What's Important by Eve Rodsky.
Evidence Based Birth Pocket Guide to Interventions by
    Rebecca Dekker PhD, RN.
The Birth Deck: 50 Ways to Comfort a Woman in Labor by Sara Lyon.

Books

"Working and Breastfeeding Made Simple" by Nancy Mohrbacher.
"Battling Over Birth Black Women And The Maternal Health Care
    Crisis" by Julie Chineyere Oparah, Helen Arega, Donitia Hudson,
    Linda Jones, and Talita Oseguera.
"Feeding the Postpartum Family with Love: Cookbook" by
    Aurella "KayBee" Kahaillia Beach.
"Visualizations for an Easier Childbirth" by Carl Jones.
"My Plus Size Pregnancy Guide Audiobook" by Jen McLellan.

"Breastfeeding Made Simple Seven Natural Laws for Nursing Mothers"
by Nancy Mohrbacher and Kathleen A. Kendall-Tackett.
"Breastfeeding Doesn't Need to Suck: How to Nurture Your Baby and
Your Mental Health" by Kathleen Kendall-Tackett.
"A Parent's Guide to a Safer Childbirth" by Gina C. Mundy J.D.
"The Mama Natural Week-by-Week Guide to Pregnancy and Childbirth"
by Genevieve Howland.
"Your Perfect Nursery" by Naomi Coe.
"Feed the Baby: An Inclusive Guide to Nursing, Bottle-Feeding and
Everything in Between by Victoria Facelli, IBCLC.
"Natural Hospital Birth: The Best of Both Worlds" by Cynthia Gabriel.
"Green Body Green Birth" by Mary Oscategui.
"Intentional Motherhood: Who Said it Would be Easy" by
Monique Russell.
"How to Raise Perfectly Imperfect Kids and Be Okay With It: Real Tips
and Strategies for Parents of Today's Gen Z Kids" by Lisa Sugarman
with Debra Fox Gansenberg, MSW, LICSW
"Real Food For Pregnancy" by Lily Nichols, RDN, CDE.
"Real Food for Gestational Diabetes" by Lily Nichols, RDN, CDE.
"The New Mommy Plan" by Valerie Lynn.
"The Mommy Plan Recipe Book" by Valerie Lynn.
"The Grace in Grief: Healing and Hope After Miscarriage" by
Laura Fletcher
"The First Forty Days The Essential Art of Nourishing the New Mother"
by Heng Ou.
"Welcome to Fatherhood" by David Arrell.
"The Birth Partner" by Penny Simkin with Katie Rohs.
"Your Amazing Newborn" by Marshall H. Klaus, MD, and
Phyllis H. Klaus, C.S.W., M.F.C.C.
"Reclaiming Postpartum Wellness: A holistic guide to returning to
the roots of health in Motherhood" by Maranda Bower.
"And Baby Makes More: Known Donors, Queer Parents and
Our Unexpected Families" by Susan Goldberg and
Chloë Brushwood Rose.

"Fertile Imagination: A Guide to Stretching Every Mom's Superpower for Maximum Impact" by Melissa Llarena.

"Fair Play: A Game-Changing Solution for When You Have Too Much to Do (and More Life to Live) by Eve Rodsky

"The Pelvic Floor: Everything You Needed to Know Sooner" by Chantal Traub, Emma Bromley, and Dr. Juan Michelle Martin.

"Birth, Breath, and Death: Meditations on Motherhood, Chaplaincy, and Life as a Doula" by Amy Wright Glenn.

"Having Twins" by Elizabeth Noble.

"Sacred Pregnancy" by Anni Daulter.

Streaming Sites

Informed Pregnancy + www.informedpregnancy.tv

Foundations and Nonprofits

Hello Seven Foundation www.helloseven.org
The Preeclampsia Foundation www.preeclampsia.org
The Colette Louise Tisdahl Foundation www.colettelouise.com/
Every Mother Counts www.everymothercounts.org
Mama Glow Foundation www.mamaglowfoundation.org
Black Mamas Matter Alliance www.blackmamasmatter.org

Maternity Leave Preparation

The Park www.theparkconsulting.com
Popins www.popinsfam.com
Chamber of Mothers www.chamberofmothers.com
The MAMAttorney www.themamattorney.com
Pumpspotting www.pumpspotting.com

Milk Storage and Donation

Milk Stork www.milkstork.com Breastmilk shipping
MILKworx www.mammaway.com Breastmilk storage products

Mother's Milk Bank www.mothersmilk.org

HumanMilk4Humanbabies www.hmbana.org

Meal Trains and Postpartum Meal Delivery Service

Take Them A Meal www.takethemameal.com

Meal Train www.mealtrain.com

Moms Meals www.momsmeals.com

Sakara www.sakara.com

Give InKind www.giveinkind.com

Mental Health Resources, contributed by Cristina Stauffer, LMSW

Postpartum Support International (PSI)

www.postpartum.net

PSI Helpline: 1-800-944-4773

Text "Help" to 800-944-4773 (English)

Text en Español: 971-203-7773

Find listings for local and online support groups, specialized therapists, and treatment centers by geographical location. Reach the PSI coordinator for your region to gain access to more treatment options. Resources for moms, dads, families, and professionals.

National Maternal Mental Health Hotline (U.S. only)

1-833-943-5746

1-833-9-HEP4MOMS

https://mchb.hrsa.gov/national-maternal-mental-health-hotline

24/7, free, confidential hotline for pregnant and new parents in English and Spanish, Interpreter Services in 60 languages, culturally sensitive support

988 Suicide and Crisis Lifeline

www.988lifeline.com

Call or text 988

Provides 24/7, free and confidential support for people in distress, prevention and crisis resources for you or your loved ones, and best practices for professionals. Local referrals provided. English, Spanish, and Deaf/Hard of Hearing options available.

Psychology Today
www.psychologytoday.com
Find a therapist with specialized training by searching by zip code and clinical specialty.

Postpartum Progress
www.postpartumprogress.com
Articles, resources and support to help understand PMAD from women who have experienced it themselves.

Books on Mental Health, contributed by Cristina Stauffer, LMSW

"This Isn't What I Expected: Overcoming Postpartum Depression" by Karen Kleiman and Valerie Davis Raskin M.D.

"Beyond the Blues: Understanding and Treating Prenatal and Postpartum Depression and Anxiety" by Shoshana S. Bennett, PhD and Pec Indman, PA, EdD

"Dropping the Baby and Other Scary Thoughts" by Karen Kleiman

"Good Moms Have Scary Thoughts: A Healing Guide to the Secret Fears of New Mothers" by Karen Kleiman, Illustrated by Molly McIntyre

"The Postpartum Partner: Practical Solutions for Living with Postpartum Depression" by Karen Kleiman (*formerly published as The Postpartum Husband - same great information but recently updated to be more inclusive of all families)

"Tokens of Affection: Reclaiming your Marriage After Postpartum Depression" by Karen Kleiman and Amy Wenzel

"What About Us? A New Parents Guide to Safeguarding Your Over-Anxious, Over-Extended, Sleep-Deprived Relationship" by Karen Kleiman, Illustrated by Molly McIntyre

"The Pregnancy and Postpartum Anxiety Workbook: Practical Skills
to Help You Overcome Anxiety, Worry, Panic Attacks, Obsessions,
and Compulsions" by Pamela S. Wiegartz, Kevin L. Gyoerkoe, et al.
"Hale's Medications and Mothers' Milk 2023: A Manual of Lactational
Pharmacology" by Thomas W. Hale, PhD
"Moods in Motion: A Coloring and Healing Book for Postpartum Moms"
by Karen Kleiman and Lisa Powell Braun
"Breathe, Mama, Breathe: 5-minute Mindfulness for Busy Moms" by
Shonda Moralis, MSW, LCSW

Nutrition

Athena's Bump www.athenasbump.com Customized nutrition for you
and baby with recipes based on your needs.

Pregnancy Subscription Boxes

Rumbly www.rumbly.co
Bump Boxes www.bumpboxes.com

Push Presents

Mrs. Push www.mrs.push.com

Vaginal Birth After Cesarean (VBAC) Resources by Jenni Froment of VBAC Academy

VBAC Academy offers free downloadable resources, access to classes
and local VBAC PROs for you to meet and learn more. Follow VBAC
Academy on Instagram (@vbacacademy) for everything you need to
know about VBAC planning and research.
"Baby Got VBAC" co-authored by Jenni Froment
"Cut, Stapled and Mended: When One Woman Reclaimed Her
Body and Gave Birth on Her Own Terms After Cesarean" by
Roanna Rosewood
"Birthing from Within" by Pam England

Evidence Based Birth, visit www.evidencebasedbirth.com to check out
the evidence between common birth-related choices presented
during pregnancy and delivery.

Fertility

Fertility Rally www.fertilityrally.com
Selah Fertility www.selahfertility.com
Naturna Institute www.naturnalife.com
Elizabeth King Coaching www.elizabethking.com

Support Groups and Mom Groups

PSI: Postpartum Support International www.postpartum.net
Breastfeeding www.lalecheleague.org
Return to Zero: H.O.P.E. www.rtzhope.org
Black Moms Connection www.blackmomsconnection.com
Dad Support www.postpartum.net/get-help/help-for-dads/
Hey Mama www.heymama.co Membership based professional
networking group for moms. They have connecting groups on
parenting and pregnancy and fertility.
MOPS International www.mops.org
Motherly www.mother.ly, Online Community

Loss

PAIL Advocates www.pailadvocates.mypixieset.com
March of Dimes www.marchofdimes.org
International Stillbirth Alliance www.stillbirthalliance.org

Positioning and Body Balancing

Webster Certified Chiropractors directory www.icpa4kids.com
Spinning Babies www.spinningbabies.com
Body Ready Method www.bodyreadymethod.com
Marya Eddaifi Coaching www.maryaeddaifi.com

Childbirth Classes

HypnoBirthing www.hypnobirthing.com
Bradley Method www.bradleybirth.com
Mama Natural www.mamnatural.com
Birth Boot Camp www.birthbootcamp.com
Gentle Birth Method www.gentlebirthmethod.com
Lamaze International www.lamaze.org
Birth and Baby University www.birthandbabyuniversity.com

Other Resources

Michael Odent www.wombecology.com
International Cesarean Awareness Network (ICAN) www.ican-online.org
American College of Obstetricians and Gynecologists (ACOG)
    www.acog.org
The Centers for Disease Control and Prevention (CDC) www.cdc.gov

Kelly Mom www.kellymom.org for breastfeeding information
American Academy of Pediatrics (AAP) www.aap.org
Healthy Children www.healthychildren.org
U.S. Consumer Product Safety Commission (CPSC) www.cpsc.gov
Motherly www.mother.ly

About the Authors

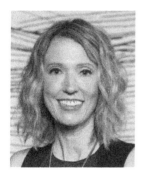

Kristin Revere, MM, CED-L, CED-PIC, NCS

Kristin is a writer, birth educator, and advocate for women's empowerment. Her passion for supporting other women has been a constant thread throughout her life, both personal and professionally. With a strong belief in the power of women, Kristin has dedicated herself to drawing out the best in those she surrounds herself with. She is the sole owner of Gold Coast Doulas.

Before discovering her love for birth work, Kristin worked as a political and nonprofit fundraiser, helping candidates raise money and fundraising for a Women's Business Center. She started her journey as a birth educator through Sacred Pregnancy in 2013 and then went on to certify with Sacred Doula and then ProDoula. Kristin is also a Certified Elite Postpartum and Infant Care Doula through ProDoula, and a Certified Transformational Birth Coach through Birth Coach Method. She is a proud Newborn Care Specialist through Newborn Care Solutions. Kristin's commitment to women's health and wellbeing is reflected in her work as a Pregnancy and Infant Loss (PAIL) Advocate and a Certified VBAC Academy Pro. Kristin launched Gold Coast Doulas in 2015 with her former business partner after owning a solo doula business.

As a Certified Gift Registry Expert through Be Her Village, Kristin has a unique perspective on supporting new parents as they prepare for their journey into parenthood. She co-hosts the Ask the Doulas podcast with Alyssa, and they co-created the Becoming A Mother online course.

Kristin earned a Bachelor of Science (BS) degree in Journalism with a minor in Political Science from Central Michigan University and a Master of Management (M.M.) in Marketing from Aquinas College. Her contributions to the community have been recognized with numerous awards including being named the #1 Birth Doula through GRKIDS in 2018, being an ATHENA Young Professional finalist multiple times through the Grand Rapids Chamber of Commerce and being named one of the 50 Most Influential Women in West Michigan by the Grand Rapids Business Journal in 2016 and 2022.

Kristin's work has been published in *First Time Parent* magazine and in *Rapid Growth*. She has had speaking engagements at multiple expos and conferences.

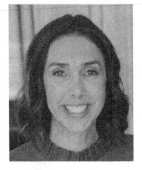

Alyssa Veneklase, CED-PIC, NCS

Alyssa Veneklase left corporate America to pursue a career as a doula a couple years after the birth of her daughter. She became passionate about supporting parents, particularly mothers, during one of the most vulnerable and trying times of their lives.

Alyssa became a Certified Elite Postpartum and Infant Care Doula in 2015. She then became a Newborn Care Specialist through Newborn Care Solutions. Alyssa is also a graduate of Advanced Multiples Training with Mama's Best Friend, a Mothership Certified Health Provider, a safeTALK Suicide Awareness Helper, and holds an Infant Safe Sleep Certificate through the Michigan Department of Health and Human Services.

She has been voted as a top postpartum doula by GRKIDS multiple times while she was a practicing doula. She was voted #1 Postpartum Doula by GRKIDs in 2018. Alyssa was an ATHENA Young Professional Finalist in 2017 through the Grand Rapids Chamber of Commerce. Alyssa was also honored with the Mom's Bloom Health Professional of the Year award in 2018. She has been published by *First Time Parent Magazine*.

Alyssa has a bachelor's degree in management from Cornerstone University and an associate's degree in liberal arts with a focus on photography from Grand Rapids Community College.

Alyssa is the former co-owner of Gold Coast Doulas. Currently she works as a licensed Real Estate Agent, supporting people through a different life transition, buying, and selling a home. She continues to teach classes and blog for Gold Coast Doulas. Alyssa co-hosts Ask the Doulas with Kristin and co-created the "Becoming A Mother" course.

About Gold Coast Doulas

Gold Coast Doulas is a birth and postpartum doula agency located in Grand Rapids, Michigan. It also serves Northern and SW Michigan lakeshore cities. The firm was established in 2015 and was the first doula agency in the area. They offer virtual and in-person services and classes. Gold Coast is a proud Certified B Corporation and won the Top Woman Owned Business in 2021 at the Grand Rapids Chamber of Commerce Epic Awards. They also received the Best of MichBusiness award in 2022.

www.goldcoastdoulas.com

About the 'Becoming A Mother' Course

Alyssa and Kristin created the self-paced birth and baby prep course called Becoming A Mother in 2020 to offer virtual support from conception through the first year. This book is based on the course. Becoming also includes live coaching calls, direct email access to Kristin and Alyssa, expert videos and a supportive community of mothers.

www.thebecomingcourse.com/join/

About Ask the Doulas Podcast

Ask the Doulas podcast launched in 2017 and is co-hosted by Alyssa and Kristin. The weekly podcast interviews experts in pregnancy, birth and early parenting. It was named one of the top 15 doula podcasts by Feedspot in 2022 and ranked #4 in the Top 100 Indie Pregnancy All Time Chart by Goodpods in 2023.

www.askthedoulas.net

Acknowledgments

Many thanks to all the amazing individuals who made this book possible.

Thank you to our students and clients who shared their personal birth and early parenting stories with us. Your raw and real experiences will help guide so many women on their journeys to motherhood.

We would also like to express our appreciation to the expert contributors for sharing their wisdom. And to our publisher Praeclarus Press for supporting our vision for this project. Ken Tackett, you have been a dream to work with. Thank you for designing the beautiful cover.

Special thanks go out to our editor Patrick Revere and to Julie Skripka for proofing the book from the lens of a mother and doula. Katherine Steffy for her research and mentoring on insurance coverage for doulas. We also want to thank Bird+Bird Photography for taking most photos you see in this book, and for capturing our team since Gold Coast launched.

This book came to life because of the *Becoming A Mother* course that Emily Richett helped us launch and promote. Thank you to Sam Veneklase, Jackie Viscusi, Jennifer Moreau, Kristie Cooley, Laura Quartey, and Kelly Peterson for your work on everything from social media, course management, podcasts, to budgeting for our various projects. Cheers to Cody Knott of Bear Productions LLC for our amazing course videos. Thanks goes out to Ben Zito of Centennial Sound for recording our audiobook.

Many thanks to our EOS Implementor Laurel Romanella, Dr. Annie Bishop and Dr. Rachel Babbitt of Rise Wellness Chiropractic PLC, B Corporation for the belief that business can be a force for good. Thanks to Marissa Berghorst at Ecobuns Baby + Co., and Mark and Emily Tobin at Hopscotch Children's Store for your constant support. Special thanks to David Arrell, author of *Welcome to Fatherhood*, and Valerie Lynn, author of *The New Mommy Plan* for endorsing *Supported*. Huge thanks to Dr. Elliot Berlin of Informed Pregnancy Project for writing the foreward to our book. Your belief in this project means the world to us.

To the nonprofits, foundations and advocacy groups making change in the maternal and infant care space, thank you. Your work is so important. We also want to recognize the legislators who sponsor and support bills like the Black Maternal Health Momnibus Act of 2021 and the PUMP for Nursing Mothers Act.

Finally, thanks to the amazing individuals who make up the birth and baby dream team, including every nurse, physician, midwife, lactation consultant, childbirth and parenting educator, birth doula, postpartum doula, antepartum doula, bereavement doula, newborn care specialist, nanny, surrogate, chiropractor, acupuncturist, sleep consultant, baby registry expert, fertility clinic, physical therapist, speech pathologist, ultrasound technician, pelvic floor therapist, prenatal massage therapist, pediatric dentist, mental health therapist, naturopathic doctor, functional medicine doctor, nutritionist, dietician, birth and newborn photographer, prenatal yoga instructor, fitness professional, car seat safety technician, baby store owner, and more. We are inspired by your dedication and passion for supporting families during this important time.

Citations

1. (n.d.). Access Denied. www.theknot.com

2. *Maternal and newborn care in the United States - Birth settings in America - NCBI bookshelf.* (2020, February 6). National Center for Biotechnology Information. www.ncbi.nlm.nih.gov/books/NBK555484/

3. (n.d.). American College of Nurse-Midwives. www.midwife.org

4. (2023, August 25). Mana. www.mana.org

5. *What is osteopathic medicine?.* (2022, January 19). American Osteopathic Association. osteopathic.org/what-is-osteopathic-medicine/

6. *Epidural versus non-epidural or no analgesia for pain management in labour.* (n.d.). PubMed Central (PMC). www.ncbi.nlm.nih.gov/pmc/articles/PMC6494646/

7. *Nytimes.com.* (n.d.). The New York Times - Breaking News, US News, World News and Videos. www.nytimes.com/article/unmedicated-birth

8. (2023, November 6). Home. www.asahq.org

9. (n.d.). Evidence Based Birth®. www.evidencebasedbirth.com/evidence-on-inducing-labor-for-going-past-your-due-date/ www.evidencebasedbirth.com/evidence-on-inducing-labor-for-going-past-your-due-date/

10. (n.d.). Evidence Based Birth®. www.evidencebasedbirth.com/evidence-for-induction-or-c-section-for-big-baby/

11. (2023, June 29). Black Mamas Matter Alliance. www.blackmamasmatter.org/12. SCOTT, K. D., KLAUS, P. H., and KLAUS, M. H. (1999). The obstetrical and postpartum benefits of continuous support during childbirth. *Journal of Women's Health and Gender-Based Medicine*, 8(10), 1257-1264. www.doi.org/10.1089/jwh.1.1999.8.1257

13. (2023, October 17). Natural Womanhood. www.naturalwomanhood.org

14. (n.d.). Cleveland Clinic. www.myclevelandclinic.org

15. (n.d.). Cleveland Clinic. www.myclevelandclinic.org

16. (n.d.). medicine.net - Medicine.net. www.medicine.net

17. (n.d.). Healthline. www.healthline.com

18. (n.d.). 403 Forbidden. www.upledger.com

19. Odent, M. (1994). *Birth reborn.* Souvenir Press.

20. *Get a car seat checked.* (n.d.). Welcome! | National CPS Certification. www.cert.safekids.org/get-car-seat-checked

21. *Lochia (Postpartum bleeding): How long, stages, smell and color.* (n.d.). Cleveland Clinic. www.my.clevelandclinic.org/health/symptoms/22485-lochia22. *Baby blues after pregnancy.* (n.d.). Help us improve the health of all moms and babies | March of Dimes. www.marchofdimes.org/find-support/topics/postpartum/baby-blues-after-pregnancy

23. *Drowsy driving.* (n.d.). NHTSA. www.nhtsa.gov/risky-driving/drowsy-driving

24. *The "short sleep" gene: When six hours is enough.* (2022, October 4). Sleep Education. www.sleepeducation.org/short-sleep-gene-when-six-hours-enough/

25. Kingshott, R. (2016, June 13). *Recharge with sleep: Pediatric sleep recommendations promoting optimal health.* American Academy of Sleep Medicine – Association for Sleep Clinicians and Researchers. www.aasm.org/recharge-with-sleep-pediatric-sleep-recommendations-promoting-optimal-health/

26. (n.d.). YouTube. www.youtube.com/watch?v=qLCq5CUqyqk

27. *4 factors that can decrease breast milk supply – and how to replenish it | Your pregnancy matters | UT southwestern Medical Center.* (n.d.). UT Southwestern Medical Center | The #1 Hospital in DFW and Texas*. www.utswmed.org/medblog/decrease-breast-milk-supply/

28. Kingshott, R. (2016, June 13). *Recharge with sleep: Pediatric sleep recommendations promoting optimal health.* American Academy of Sleep Medicine – Association for Sleep Clinicians and Researchers. www.aasm.org/recharge-with-sleep-pediatric-sleep-recommendations-promoting-optimal-health/

Contributors

Expert Contributors

Amber Kilpatrick is a spiritual ecologist, healing centered yoga teacher, and founder of Mindful School of Yoga™. You can find her at www.mindfulyogaschool.com and www.amberkilpatrick.com

Kelly Wysocki-Emery, MSN, RN, IBCLC, is a breastfeeding educator for Gold Coast Doulas and the owner of Baby beloved, Inc. Kelly has been helping mothers breastfeed since 1994. She works in private practice as well as for a hospital system, and splits her time between the hospital, six pediatric offices, and private home consultations. She also teaches breastfeeding classes through Gold Coast as well as virtually and in-person through Baby beloved, Inc, which she loves. Kelly breastfed two babies, and it was those babies who changed her trajectory in life to become a lactation consultant. www.babybeloved.com

Cristina Stauffer, LMSW, is a psychotherapist who owns her own private practice in Grand Rapids, MI. Cristina earned a Bachelor of Arts degree in psychology from the University of Michigan and a master's in social work degree from Boston University. She has practiced in the field of maternal mental health for over 25 years. Cristina believes in a relationship-based approach to therapy meaning that it is important to her to establish a place of trust, mutual respect, support, and healing with her clients. Her passions include supporting women and families through adjustment to pregnancy and early parenthood, perinatal mood and anxiety disorders including postpartum depression, complicated pregnancy, traumatic birth, infertility, miscarriage and infant loss, medically fragile infants, infant mental health, and bonding and attachment. Cristina is also a Certified Educator of Infant Massage (CEIM). When not at work, Cristina enjoys reading, yoga, crafting and spending time with her husband and her two daughters.

Angela Tallon, M.D., is our expert contributor to the newborn procedures chapter. Dr. Tallon is a pediatrician practicing in Grand Haven, Michigan. In addition to her experience in general pediatrics, she also has experience in the field of child abuse and neglect medicine. Dr. Tallon lives in Allendale with her husband and their six daughters. She has always wanted to be an author in any capacity and hopes to pursue writing later in her career.

Heidi McDowell is the Owner of Mind Body Baby, a specialty Yoga and Barre studio in Grand Rapids, Michigan and is a former birth and postpartum doula with Gold Coast Doulas. Heidi is a Yoga Alliance E-RYT, a Registered Prenatal Yoga Teacher, Certified Barre Instructor, Labor Doula, a Body Ready Method Pro, and has taken trainings with Yoga Teacher Jason Crandall and Gail Tully of Spinning Babies.

Jenni Froment has been teaching parents and professionals about VBAC birth since 2013, after her own VBA2C birth experience created a passion in her for helping others achieve VBAC. She spent four years as the chapter leader of a local VBAC advocacy and support group, called ICAN of Phoenix, before beginning her career as a self-proclaimed, "VBAC Doula". In 2016, she was trained and certified as a professional doula and started accepting doula clients. Since then, she has specialized in supporting VBAC births and has served hundreds of VBAC clients through support groups, community service and her doula work. In 2020, she launched VBAC Academy and now her focus is on increasing access to VBAC through online classes and easy to access VBAC content on social media. VBAC Academy offers professional, evidence-based training for parents and professionals. Jenni has had one emergency cesarean, one planned cesarean, one VBA2C with an epidural and one unmedicated VBA2C. She lives in Phoenix, AZ with husband and kids.

Lizzie Williams helps teams and organizations build community and connection through creative experiences, thoughtful communication, and values-based strategic alignment. She lives with her husband, their daughter, and her two teenage stepsons in Grand Rapids, Michigan.

Katherine Steffy, MPH, is a healthcare management professional with a decade+ of educational leadership, strategic planning, and operations experience. She also owns and operates a consultancy, KS Insights.

Birth and Baby Story Contributors

We can't thank our contributors enough for sharing their personal birth and parenting journeys with our readers: Lindsay Carlson, Liz Waid, Elise Slade, Lexi Zuyddyk, Sasha Wolff, Katie Dykema, Samantha Veneklase, Meagen Coburn, Marta Johnson-Ebels, Tabetha Thomas, Dr. Rachel Babbitt, Lizzie Williams, Bri Luginbill, and Dominique Tol.

External References

Exercise by Heidi McDowell

Exercise During Pregnancy. (2019, July). The American College of Obstetricians and Gynecologists. www.acog.org/womens-health/faqs/exercise-during-pregnancy

National Center for Health Statistics. Health, United States, 2013: With Special Feature on Prescription Drugs. Hyattsville, MD. 2014. www.cdc.gov/nchs/data/hus/hus13.pdf#068

Newborn Procedures

Baskin MD. Patient education: Circumcision in baby boys (Beyond the Basics)

Lockwood C; Wilcox D, ed. UpToDate. Waltham, MA: UpToDate Inc. www.uptodate.com (Accessed on June 29, 2019.)

Drutz MD. Hepatitis B virus immunization in infants, children, and adolescents. Duryea T; Edwards M, ed. UpToDate. Waltham, MA: UpToDate Inc. www.uptodate.com (Accessed on June 28, 2019.)

Isaacson MD. Ankyloglossia (tongue-tie) in infants and children. Messner A, ed. UpToDate. Waltham, MA: UpToDate Inc. www.uptodate.com (Accessed on June 28, 2019.)

McKee-Garrett MD. Overview of the routine management of the healthy newborn infant. Weisman L, ed. UpToDate. Waltham, MA: UpToDate Inc. www.uptodate.com (Accessed on June 28, 2019.)

Pazirandeh MD et al. Overview of vitamin K. Seres D; Motil K, ed. UpToDate. Waltham, MA: UpToDate Inc. www.uptodate.com (Accessed on June 28, 2019.)

Speer MD. Gonococcal infection in the newborn. Weisman L; Kaplan S, ed. UpToDate. Waltham, MA: UpToDate Inc. www.uptodate.com (Accessed on June 28, 2019.)

Maternal Health and Mortality

Evidence Based Birth (http://evidencebasedbirth.com/the-evidence-for-doulas/)

Hodenett, Gates, Hofmeyr, Sakala. Continuous support for women during childbirth (http://www.ncbi.nlm.nih.gov/pubmed/23076901)

Safe Prevention of the Primary Cesarean Delivery. American Congress of Obstetricians and Gynecologists. 2014. (http://www.acog.org/Resources-And-Publications/Obstetric-Care-Consensus-Series/Safe-Prevention-of-the-Primary-Cesarean-Delivery)

Kozhimannil, KB. Doula care, birth outcomes, and costs among Medicaid beneficiaries. 2013. American Journal of Public Health (http://www.ncbi.nlm.nih.gov/m/pubmed/23409910/)

Doulas ease stress, increase satisfaction with birthing experience, statistics indicate. 2014. (http://www.sciencedaily.com/releases/2014/03/140305124943.htm)

Kozhimannil K and Hardeman R. How Medicaid Coverage for Doula Care Could Improve Birth Outcomes, Reduce Costs, and Improve Equity. 2014. Health Affairs. (http://healthaffairs.org/blog/2015/07/01/how-medicaid-coverage-for-doula-care-could-improve-birth-outcomes-reduce-costs-and-improve-equity/)

Gruber, Cupito and Dobson. Impact of Doulas on Healthy Birth Outcomes. 2013. Journal of Perinatal Education. (http://www.ncbi.nlm.nih.gov/pmc/articles/PMC3647727/)

Interview with Kristin Revere, doula and owner of Gold Cost Doulas. September 17, 2015.

Kozhimannil, KB, Law, Michael R., and Virning, Beth A. Cesarean Delivery Rates Very Tenfold Among US Hospitals; Reducing Variation Mat Address Quality And Cost Issues. Health Affairs 32, no. 3 (2013):527-535

Kozhimannil, KB, Macheras, Michelle, Lorch, Scott A. Trends in Childbirth Before 39 Weeks' Gestation without Medical Indication. Med Care. 2014 July; 52(7): 649-657.

Kozhimannil, Hardeman, Alarid-Escudero, Vogelsang, Blauer-Peterson, and Howell. Modeling the Cost-Effectiveness of Doula Care Associated with Reductions in Preterm Birth and Cesarean Delivery. Birth 43:1, March 2016. (www.onlinelibrary.wiley.com/doi/full/10.1111/birt.12218)

Research/Project for the purposes of developing doula benefit. Priority Health, Grand Rapids, Michigan. 2015-2018.

Artiga S, Pham O, Orgera K, Ranji U. Racial Disparities in Maternal and Infant Health: An Overview. Kaiser Family Foundation. November 10, 2020. Dekker, Rebecca. Evidence on: doulas. Evidence Based Birth. www.evidencebasedbirth.com/the-evidence-for-doulas/ May 4, 2019.

Murphy, Carrie. Midwives are growing in popularity. Here's what you need to know. Healthline. www.healthline.com/health/midwives-growing-in-popularity-what-to-know October 31, 2018.

Haelle, Tara. Doula Support for Pregnant Women Could Improve Care, Reduce Costs. National Public Radio. www.npr.org/sections/health-shots/2016/01/15/463223250/doula-support-for-pregnant-women-could-improve-care-reduce-costs. January 15, 2016.

Preliminary study presented to the American Congress of Obstetricians and Gynecologists.

American Journal of Public Health. 2013.
American Academy of Pediatrics

Journal of Obstetric, Gynecologic, and Neonatal Nursing. 2009.

Lender, Paul. How Plans Can Improve Outcomes and Cut Costs for Preterm Infant Care. Managed Care Mag.com. www.managedcaremag.com/archives/2010/1/how-plans-can-improve-outcomes-and-cut-costs-preterm-infant-care/. 2010.

Muraskas MD, Jonathan, Parsi JD PhD, Kayhan. The Cost of Saving the Tiniest Lives: NICUs versus Prevention. AMA Journal of Ethics. www.journalofethics.ama-assn.org/article/cost-saving-tiniest-lives-nicus-versus-prevention/2008-10. October 2008.

Journal of Occupational and Environmental Medicine, 2012.

Journal of Women's Health and Gender Based Medicine, 1999.

Gjerdingen, Dwenda Kay et al. Doula and Peer Telephone Support for Postpartum Depression: A pilot randomized controlled trial. Journal of Primary Care and Community Health. www.journals.sagepub.com/doi/full/10.1177/2150131912451598. June 2012.

Made in the USA
Monee, IL
07 June 2024

59561500R00128